Theory & Practice of Therapeutic Massage Exam Review, 5th Edition

Mark F. Beck

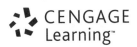
CENGAGE
Learning™

Australia • Brazil • Japan • Korea • Mexico • Singapore • Spain • United Kingdom • United States

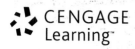
CENGAGE
Learning™

Theory & Practice of Therapeutic Massage Exam Review

Edition: 5

Author(s): Mark F. Beck

President, Milady: Dawn Gerrain

Publisher: Erin O'Connor

Acquisitions Editor: Martine Edwards

Senior Product Manager: Philip Mandl

Editorial Assistant: Maria Herbert

Director of Beauty Industry Relations: Sandra Bruce

Executive Marketing Manager: Gerard McAvey

Production Director: Wendy Troeger

Senior Content Project Manager: Angela Sheehan

Senior Art Director: Joy Kocsis

For product information and technology assistance, contact us at
Professional & Career Group Customer Support, 1-800-648-7450

For permission to use material from this text or product, submit all requests online at **cengage.com/permissions.**
Further permissions questions can be e-mailed to
permissionrequest@cengage.com.

Library of Congress Control Number: 2009938144

ISBN-13: 978-1-4354-8528-0
ISBN-10: 1-4354-8528-9

Milady
5 Maxwell Drive
Clifton Park, NY 12065-2919
USA

Cengage Learning products are represented in Canada by Nelson Education, Ltd.

For your lifelong learning solutions, visit
milady.cengage.com

Visit our corporate website at **cengage.com.**

Notice to the Reader
Publisher does not warrant or guarantee any of the products described herein or perform any independent analysis in connection with any of the product information contained herein. Publisher does not assume, and expressly disclaims, any obligation to obtain and include information other than that provided to it by the manufacturer. The reader is expressly warned to consider and adopt all safety precautions that might be indicated by the activities described herein and to avoid all potential hazards. By following the instructions contained herein, the reader willingly assumes all risks in connection with such instructions. The publisher makes no representations or warranties of any kind, including but not limited to, the warranties of fitness for particular purpose or merchantability, nor are any such representations implied with respect to the material set forth herein, and the publisher takes no responsibility with respect to such material. The publisher shall not be liable for any special, consequential, or exemplary damages resulting, in whole or part, from the readers' use of, or reliance upon, this material.

A0068356
25/4/12
£15-36
646.75

Printed in the United States of America
1 2 3 4 5   12 11 10

Theory & Practice of Therapeutic Massage Exam Review

Foreword

Theory & Practice of Therapeutic Massage, 5th Edition Exam Review follows the type of massage therapy questions most frequently used by massage therapy testing boards, conducted under the auspices of the Federation of State Massage Therapy Boards: Massage & Bodywork Licensing Examination (MBLEx), and the National Certification Board for Therapeutic Massage & Bodywork: the National Certification Examination (NCE).

This exam review book is designed to be of major assistance to students in preparing for the examinations and future career path. The exclusive concentration on multiple-choice test items reflects the fact that most certification and licensing examinations are confined to this type of question.

Questions on the different examinations will not be exactly like these and may not touch upon all the information covered in this review. But students who diligently study and practice their work as taught in the classroom and who use this book for test preparation and review should receive higher grades on both classroom and license examinations.

The answers to the questions are found at the end of the book.

Part 1: The History and Advancement of Therapeutic Massage

CHAPTER 1—HISTORICAL OVERVIEW OF MASSAGE

MULTIPLE CHOICE

1. In the past, a female massage practitioner was called a:
   a. massager
   b. masseur
   c. masseuse
   d. masso _____

2. The Sanskrit term _____ means to press softly.
   a. *makeh*
   b. *massa*
   c. *mass'h*
   d. *masso* _____

3. In the United States, the use of the word *massage* was popularized by:
   a. Herodicus
   b. Douglas Graham
   c. Aesculapius
   d. Johann Georg Mezger _____

4. Massage has been important in Western medical traditions for at least _____ years.
   a. 5,000
   b. 3,000
   c. 2,000
   d. 1,000 _____

5. A modern term for Chinese massage is:
   a. *anmo*
   b. *tschanpua*
   c. *tsubo*
   d. *tui-na* _____

6. The Japanese term for energy point or pressure point is:
   a. Ayurveda
   b. Tsai
   c. tschanpua
   d. tsubo _____

7. _____ is a Japanese finger-pressure massage technique.
   a. Shiatsu
   b. Tapotement
   c. Tsubo
   d. *Tui-na* _____

8. _____ is a Hindu technique of massage in the bath.
   a. Anmo
   b. Shiatsu
   c. Tschanpua
   d. Tsubo _____

9. In his writings, Hippocrates used the word _____, which means the art of rubbing a body part upward.
   a. *anatripsis*
   b. *Ayurveda*
   c. *Hippocratic*
   d. *tschanpua*
   ____

10. William Harvey, an English physician, is credited with discovering _____ in 1628.
    a. anatripsis
    b. blood circulation
    c. lymphedema
    d. massage
    ____

11. _____ gained great knowledge of anatomy in his role as a physician to gladiators.
    a. Cicero
    b. Galen
    c. Hippocrates
    d. Rhazes
    ____

12. Persian philosopher/physician _____ authored the *Canon of Medicine*, considered the most important book in medical history.
    a. Avicenna
    b. Galen
    c. Herodicus
    d. Rhazes
    ____

13. _____ classified massage movements as gentle, medium, and vigorous frictions and employed flexion, extension, and circumduction of joints.
    a. Avicenna
    b. Galen
    c. William Harvey
    d. Ambroise Pare
    ____

14. In 1569, _____ published *De Arte Gymnastica* on gymnastics and the benefits of massage when integrated into body and mind treatments.
    a. Galen
    b. William Harvey
    c. Mercurialis
    d. Ambroise Pare
    ____

15. In the early nineteenth century, Englishman _____ was a surgeon and practitioner of chirurgy, or healing with the hands.
    a. Douglas Graham
    b. John Grosvenor
    c. William Harvey
    d. Mathias Roth
    ____

16. _____ gymnastics, or gymnastics applied to the treatment of disease, was developed by Per Henrik Ling.
    a. Duplicated
    b. Swedish
    c. Medical
    d. Tapotement
    ____

17. In the Ling System, _____ movements are performed by the patient and can be called exercise.
    a. active
    b. duplicated
    c. passive
    d. therapeutic
    ____

18. Mathias Roth, an English physician, published the first English book on the Swedish Movements in:
    a. 1813
    b. 1851
    c. 1858
    d. 1861 ____

19. Modern massage terminology is credited to:
    a. Johann Mezger
    b. Mathias Roth
    c. Charles Fayette Taylor
    d. Emil Vodder ____

20. In massage, _____ lifts, squeezes, and presses the tissues.
    a. effleurage
    b. friction
    c. petrissage
    d. tapotement ____

21. _____ is a succession of strokes applied by gliding the hand over an extended portion of the body.
    a. Effleurage
    b. Friction
    c. Petrissage
    d. Tapotement ____

22. Albert J. Hoffa's _____, one of the most basic books in the field of massage, contains many of the techniques used in Swedish massage.
    a. *Art of Massage*
    b. *Good Health*
    c. *Healing Massage Techniques*
    d. *Technik Der Massage* ____

23. The invention of _____ had a detrimental effect on hands-on massage therapy.
    a. computers
    b. electricity
    c. lymphatics
    d. spas ____

24. Emil Vodder developed _____, a method of gentle rhythmical massage that effectively treats chronic lymphedema.
    a. connective tissue massage
    b. Esalen massage
    c. lymphatics
    d. manual lymph drainage ____

25. Which one of the following massage types is believed to affect vascular and visceral reflexes related to varied pathologies and disabilities?
    a. Connective Tissue Massage
    b. Deep Transverse Friction Massage
    c. Esalen Massage
    d. Manual Lymph Drainage ____

26. _____, an English orthopedic physician, is credited with popularizing Deep Transverse Friction Massage.
    a. James H. Cyriax
    b. Elizabeth Dicke
    c. Maria Ebner
    d. Emil Vodder ____

27. Beginning around _____, a massage renaissance that continues today began in the United States.
    a. 1950   c. 1970
    b. 1960   d. 1980   ____

28. The Esalen Institute in Big Sur California, founded in 1962, became a popular center for which of the following?
    a. human potential movement   c. Trager method
    b. preventive health movement   d. wellness model   ____

29. Which of the following is the oldest national professional massage association in the United States?
    a. ABMP   c. AOBTA
    b. AMTA   d. IMA   ____

30. The National Certification Exam, established in 1990, required applicants to have at least _____ hours of training from a state-recognized school.
    a. 100   c. 800
    b. 500   d. 1,000   ____

31. _____ massage is designed to enhance athletes' performances.
    a. Deep tissue   c. Sports
    b. Chair   d. Team   ____

32. _____ massage was a great innovation that helped demystify massage and make it more accessible to a wider audience.
    a. Chair   c. Sports
    b. Floor   d. Table   ____

33. By 2009, _____ states and the District of Columbia had state-wide massage licensing.
    a. 10   c. 30
    b. 20   d. 40   ____

34. In 2005, the _____ was established when members from twenty-two state massage therapy licensing agencies convened.
    a. APTA   c. NCBTMB
    b. FSMTB   d. NCE   ____

4

35. In 1992, Tiffany M. Fields founded the _____ in
collaboration with the University of Miami Medical School.
a. Center for Complementary and   c. National Institutes
     Alternative Medicine   of Health
b. Massage Therapy Foundation   d. Touch Research Institute   ____

36. In 1998, the NIH established the:
a. AMTA   c. NCCAM
b. CAM   d. TRI   ____

37. Which system of massage stems from the Chinese medical practice
of acupuncture?
a. acupressure   c. Swedish
b. shiatsu   d. tsubo   ____

38. Shiatsu, a finger pressure method, is based on the Oriental
concept that the body has a series of energy points called:
a. *chi*   c. *tui-na*
b. *Ki*   d. tsubo   ____

39. Which massage system is said to improve body metabolism and
relieve a number of physical disorders?
a. acupressure   c. Japanese
b. German   d. Swedish   ____

40. _____ is a method developed by Randolph Stone that uses
massage manipulations derived from both Eastern and Western
practices.
a. Polarity therapy   c. Sports massage
b. Rolfing   d. Trager method   ____

41. _____ aligns the major body segments through
manipulation of the connective tissue.
a. Polarity therapy   c. Rolfing
b. Reflexology   d. Trager method   ____

42. _____ stimulates particular points on the surface of the
body, which in turn affect other body areas or organs.
a. Craniosacral therapy   c. Touch for Health
b. Reflexology   d. Trager method   ____

43. _____ is a simplified form of applied kinesiology that
involves techniques from both Eastern and Western origins.
a. Neuromuscular technique   c. Rolfing
b. Reflexology   d. Touch for Health   ____

44. Around 1940, osteopaths Stanley Lief and Boris Chaitow originated: _____
    a. neuromuscular techniques   c. Rolfing
    b. reflexology   d. Trager method   ____

45. John Upledger is credited with developing which of the following?
    a. craniosacral therapy   c. neuromuscular
                                        techniques
    b. kinesiology   d. reflexology   ____

CHAPTER 2—REQUIREMENTS FOR THE PRACTICE OF THERAPEUTIC MASSAGE

MULTIPLE CHOICE

1. The massage practitioner has an ethical responsibility to the public and to:
   a. other businesses
   b. clients
   c. insurance companies
   d. no answers
   _____

2. According to law, who can diagnose illnesses and other medical conditions and prescribe medications for those conditions?
   a. doctors
   b. doctors and registered nurses
   c. nurse's aides
   d. pharmacists
   _____

3. An individual's scope of practice is directly related to _____ and _____.
   a. clients, training
   b. skills, training
   c. ethics, clients
   d. beliefs, skills
   _____

4. Many occupations and professions have national or state regulatory boards that help define and enforce adherence to a(n):
   a. ethical practice
   b. rule of business
   c. scope of practice
   d. standard of practice
   _____

5. Which of the following statements about scope of practice is *not* true?
   a. Personal bias influences a person's scope of practice.
   b. Educational focus influences a practitioner's scope of practice.
   c. Scope of practice is influenced by the skills acquired.
   d. Massage therapy has a clearly defined scope of practice.
   _____

6. In the United States, _____ percent of states have adopted licensing regulations for massage practice.
   a. 40
   b. 60
   c. 80
   d. 90
   _____

7. Many municipalities adopt ordinances to curb unethical practices and use of the term _____ to conceal questionable or illegal activities.
   a. *license*
   b. *massage*
   c. *municipal*
   d. *practice*
   _____

8. Ordinances adopted to curb unethical and illegal practices in massage practice include all of the following *except*:
   a. criminal record searches
   b. fingerprinting
   c. mug shots
   d. proficiency exams _____

9. A massage license from a city is most likely valid:
   a. only in the city where issued
   b. throughout the state where issued
   c. only in the county where issued
   d. throughout the United States _____

10. All of the following will be able to provide information concerning massage regulations *except*:
    a. city attorney
    b. county commissioner's office
    c. department of health
    d. mayor's office _____

11. _____ between two licensing entities means that the two entities will honor a valid massage license.
    a. Dualism
    b. Grandfathering
    c. Reciprocity
    d. Statute sharing _____

12. In terms of massage licensing, which laws usually take precedence?
    a. city
    b. county
    c. federal
    d. state _____

13. Which of the following is *not* a requirement for state licensure?
    a. massage therapy training
    b. complete written exam
    c. high school diploma
    d. minimum 21-year age _____

14. Both NCE and MBLEx are exams in _____ format.
    a. written-essay
    b. multiple-choice
    c. short-answer
    d. true-false _____

15. All of the following are subjects covered on the NCE exam *except*:
    a. benefits
    b. kinesiology
    c. morphology
    d. pathology _____

16. Which of the following is a service within a massage therapist's scope of practice?
    a. acupuncture
    b. chiropractic assessment
    c. psychotherapy
    d. therapeutic assessment _____

17. When setting up a massage practice, local business and
_____ laws must be followed.
a. education   c. medical
b. massage   d. zoning   _____

18. COMTA requires schools to have at least _____ classroom
hours of training before consideration for accreditation.
a. 500   c. 800
b. 600   d. 1,000   _____

19. Subjects required in COMTA training include all of the
following *except*:
a. assessment, planning, and   c. effects of massage and
     performance   bodywork
b. business development   d. massage contraindications
     and practices   and precautions   _____

20. In states that license massage, educational requirements vary
from _____ to _____ hours of training.
a. 300, 600   c. 300, 1,000
b. 500, 1,000   d. 300, 2,200   _____

21. Continuing education is among the renewal requirements for all of
the following *except*:
a. ABMP   c. FSMTB
b. AMTA   d. NCB   _____

22. Which of the following is *not* a purpose of a massage therapist's
continuing education courses?
a. expand technical skills   c. improve business
b. hire employees   d. refresh interest   _____

23. Some states require a(n) _____ for licensing, which serves as
proof of the massage therapist's adequate health.
a. doctor's permission   c. insurance certificate
b. health certificate   d. physician referral   _____

24. Health requirements for the massage practitioner include
_____ and the ability to concentrate.
a. annual physical exams   c. certification
b. cardiovascular fitness   d. physical stamina   _____

25. Massage practitioners could have their licenses revoked, suspended, or canceled for any of the following reasons *except*:
    a. ethical misconduct
    b. felony conviction
    c. narcotics addiction
    d. misdemeanor conviction _____

26. Which of the following is awarded by schools and institutions to show the successful completion of a course of study?
    a. award
    b. certificate
    c. license
    d. regulation _____

27. Which of the following National Certification Board (NCB) exams focuses on classic Western massage without the Asian bodywork component?
    a. NCBTMB
    b. NCE
    c. NCETM
    d. NCETMB _____

CHAPTER 3—PROFESSIONAL ETHICS FOR MASSAGE PRACTITIONERS

MULTIPLE CHOICE

1. A profession is usually regulated, is represented by a professional association, and adheres to a:
   a. scope of practice
   b. code of ethics
   c. moral code
   d. professional strategy _____

2. Educational requirements, scopes of practice, codes of ethics, and state and local regulations are all examples of:
   a. ethical standards
   b. practical ethics
   c. professional ethics
   d. professional standards _____

3. Everyone has _____ that dictate how they act and interact with the world and other people.
   a. boundaries
   b. ethics
   c. force fields
   d. strategies _____

4. _____ provide protection and a sense of self.
   a. Moral codes
   b. Professional boundaries
   c. Personal boundaries
   d. Defense zones _____

5. _____ boundaries are predetermined practices that protect the safety of the client and the therapist.
   a. Ethical
   b. Professional
   c. Personal
   d. Physical _____

6. The eight major areas to consider when establishing professional boundaries include all of the following *except*:
   a. appearance
   b. language
   c. money
   d. self-perception _____

7. Voice intonation is a component of which type of professional boundary?
   a. appearance
   b. interpersonal space
   c. language
   d. self-disclosure _____

8. _____ refers to a therapeutic massage setting that is professional, safe, and comfortable.
   a. Location
   b. Appearance
   c. Time
   d. no answers _____

9. When first establishing interpersonal space with a client, the massage therapist should be:
   a. standing while the client sits
   b. sitting if the client is standing
   c. always standing
   d. at the client's eye level _____

10. In self-disclosure, the information needed to gain the client's informed consent and confidence includes all of the following *except*:
    a. appointment policies
    b. marital status
    c. modalities practiced
    d. treatment plan _____

11. Which of the following areas of professional boundaries relates directly to physical boundaries on and off of the table?
    a. appearance
    b. language
    c. self-disclosure
    d. touch _____

12. Touch boundaries on the treatment table include all of the following *except*:
    a. touch depth and quality
    b. supervised touch
    c. which parts of the client's body are not touched
    d. which parts of the practitioner's body touch the client _____

13. Touch that is too _____ may cause discomfort and violate boundaries.
    a. light
    b. deep
    c. light or deep
    d. neither light nor deep _____

14. Time boundaries are defined by establishing and maintaining policies regarding all of the following *except*:
    a. late arrivals
    b. late payments
    c. missed appointments
    d. session length _____

15. Fees that are too low or exorbitantly high for the services rendered are professional boundary:
    a. adjustments
    b. infractions
    c. regulations
    d. all answers _____

16. The therapeutic relationship is a practitioner/client relationship that is _____-centered.
    a. client
    b. money
    c. practitioner
    d. time _____

17. A _____ is a place where clients assume they are safe from physical, emotional, and sexual impropriety.
    a. client space
    c. safe environment
    b. massage practice
    d. treatment space
    ____

18. _____ in the practitioner/client relationship is the foundation of safety, protection, trust, and respect.
    a. Compromise
    c. Equality
    b. Confidentiality
    d. Relaxation
    ____

19. The _____ legally requires massage therapists to report situations of imminent or life-threatening danger by or to a client.
    a. confidentiality clause
    c. power differential
    b. duty to warn and protect
    d. right of client privilege
    ____

20. In a client-based relationship, the question "To whose benefit is the questioned activity?" determines:
    a. client satisfaction
    c. procedure time allotment
    b. procedure appropriateness
    d. confidential information
    ____

21. In a(n) _____ relationship, one party has more authority while the other is more vulnerable or submissive.
    a. subordinate relationship
    c. peer relationship
    b. imbalance differential
    d. power differential
    ____

22. In which of the following relationships is the power differential fairly even?
    a. husband/wife
    c. student/teacher
    b. employer/employee
    d. practitioner/client
    ____

23. A feeling of _____ can signal the crossing of a personal boundary.
    a. unease
    c. pleasure
    b. surprise
    d. pain
    ____

24. _____ is/are the most effective tool for both preventing and clarifying boundary issues.
    a. Clear communication
    c. Litigation
    b. Ethical standards
    d. Policies
    ____

25. In the therapeutic relationship, who is responsible for being sensitive to, respecting, and maintaining personal and professional boundaries?
   a. client
   b. employee
   c. practitioner
   d. no answers   ____

26. A client's unconscious tendency to project onto the practitioner the attributes of someone from a former relationship is called:
   a. transference
   b. power differential
   c. communication
   d. countertransference   ____

27. _____ tends to diminish the effectiveness of the therapeutic relationship.
   a. Communication
   b. Confidentiality
   c. Projection
   d. Transference   ____

28. It is *not* a sign of transference when the client does which of the following?
   a. demands more of the practitioner's time
   b. proposes sexual involvement
   c. berates the practitioner
   d. chooses to end treatment   ____

29. Clients who bring their practitioners gifts may be exhibiting signs of:
   a. appreciation
   b. countertransference
   c. power differential
   d. transference   ____

30. Which of the following is *not* a sign of countertransference?
   a. The client brings or offers the practitioner gifts or favors.
   b. The practitioner dreads an upcoming appointment with a client.
   c. The practitioner experiences fatigue or depression after a session.
   d. The practitioner thinks excessively about a client between sessions. ____

31. Dressing in a special manner for certain clients may be a sign of:
   a. countertransference
   b. dual relationship
   c. power differential
   d. transference   ____

32. The best defense against transference and countertransference is:
   a. abiding by state mandates
   b. discontinuing the relationship
   c. limiting services to family and close friends
   d. maintaining healthy professional boundaries   ____

33. Bartering for work or services may create what type of relationship?
    a. balance of power
    b. dual
    c. nontherapeutic
    d. power differential _____

34. Which of the following is a classic dual relationship?
    a. client barters for massage services
    b. client and practitioner take on other roles
    c. practitioner barters massage for other services
    d. client refers friends to the practitioner _____

35. The practitioner who develops feelings for a client should do which of the following?
    a. ask the client out to coffee
    b. assess the client's feelings
    c. determine mutual consent
    d. refer the client to another practitioner _____

36. Who is responsible for maintaining professional boundaries?
    a. client
    b. massage therapist
    c. peer supervisor
    d. all answers _____

37. The positive touch of massage increases which of the following?
    a. cortisol
    b. dopamine
    c. norepinephrine
    d. stress _____

38. People who suffer from depression have low levels of:
    a. cortisol
    b. epinephrine
    c. norepinephrine
    d. serotonin _____

39. Touch is considered _____ when it is applied to do harm to or dominate the receiver.
    a. aggressive
    b. casual
    c. erotic
    d. no answers _____

40. In a therapeutic setting, _____ touch is never appropriate.
    a. casual
    b. erotic
    c. positive
    d. therapeutic _____

41. _____ is a natural physiological and cognitive response to stimulation perceived as erotic by the body.
    a. Positive touch
    b. Sexual abuse
    c. Sexual arousal
    d. Touch therapy _____

42. Which of the following conceals most signs of a woman's sexual arousal?
    a. careful lighting
    b. proper draping
    c. proper table position
    d. no answers
    _____

43. Therapists who find they are involved in cases of transference, countertransference, or dual relationships should pursue:
    a. client referral
    b. power differentials
    c. supervision
    d. therapeutic massage
    _____

44. In _____ supervision, therapists who practice similar forms of therapy meet regularly and consistently using an agreed-upon format.
    a. mentor
    b. peer group
    c. mental health
    d. clinical
    _____

45. Which of the following is *not* an example of ethical standards of practice?
    a. maintaining accurate client records
    b. staying within scope of practice
    c. treating clients with courtesy
    d. sharing client information freely
    _____

46. _____ is the ability to be tolerant under stressful or undesirable conditions.
    a. Intuition
    b. Honesty
    c. Patience
    d. Tact
    _____

47. The quality of being reliable, responsible, self-disciplined, and well adjusted is:
    a. tact
    b. intuition
    c. maturity
    d. self-motivation
    _____

48. _____ is projected by attitudes about self and one's chosen profession.
    a. Cheerfulness
    b. Honesty
    c. Intuition
    d. Self-esteem
    _____

49. The ability to set positive goals and put forth the energy and effort needed to achieve those goals is called:
    a. self-motivation
    b. self-esteem
    c. tact
    d. maturity
    _____

50. A(n) _____ is particularly important in personal service because professionals address the health and well-being of individuals.
    a. appropriate business name
    b. reliable reputation
    c. robust business plan
    d. employee handbook
    _____

Part 2: Human Anatomy and Physiology

CHAPTER 4 —OVERVIEW OF HUMAN ANATOMY AND PHYSIOLOGY

MULTIPLE CHOICE

1. _____ is the science of structure of an organism or body.
   a. Anatomy
   c. Pathology
   b. Kinesiology
   d. Physiology ____

2. _____ concerns the normal functions performed by various body systems.
   a. Anatomy
   c. Pathology
   b. Kinesiology
   d. Physiology ____

3. The scientific study of muscular activity and the mechanics of body movement is called:
   a. anatomy
   c. pathology
   b. kinesiology
   d. physiology ____

4. _____ examines what happens when the body or a body part is in a state of dysfunction or disease.
   a. Anatomy
   c. Pathology
   b. Kinesiology
   d. Physiology ____

5. Reflex effects of massage include all of the following *except*:
   a. reduced heart rate
   c. deeper breathing
   b. increased local circulation
   d. slower breathing ____

6. Increased circulation to internal organs, reduced blood pressure, and general muscle relaxation are examples of _____ massage effects.
   a. indirect
   c. reflex
   b. basic
   d. direct ____

7. A basic knowledge of _____ gives massage therapists an understanding of disease processes.
   a. physiology
   c. kinesiology
   b. pathology
   d. anatomy ____

8. When the body's _____ is disturbed, a person may experience disease symptoms.
   a. blood
   c. lymph
   b. homeostasis
   d. system ____

9. _____ are observable indications of a disease.
   a. Indicators   c. Stages
   b. Signs   d. Symptoms   ____

10. Which of the following is *not* a sign of disease?
    a. fever   c. chills
    b. abnormal skin color   d. physical irregularities   ____

11. The basis for disease diagnosis includes all of the following
    except:
    a. homeostasis   c. laboratory tests
    b. symptoms and signs   d. medical histories   ____

12. Age, working or living conditions, gender, and heredity are
    _____ factors in disease.
    a. direct   c. predisposing
    b. indirect   d. stress   ____

13. _____ is any psychological or physical situation or
    condition that causes tension or strain.
    a. Disease   c. Pain
    b. Homeostasis   d. Stress   ____

14. During times of stress, _____ provide a physical and
    mental boost that heightens the senses and sharpens the reflexes.
    a. adrenal secretions   c. parasites
    b. glycogens   d. stressors   ____

15. During times of stress, all of the following glands affect the
    function of most internal systems *except* the:
    a. adrenal   c. pituitary
    b. hypothalamus   d. thyroid   ____

16. The principal and most understood adrenal hormones are
    _____ and _____.
    a. adrenaline, cortisol   c. cortisol, epinephrine
    b. prolactin, estrogen   d. epinephrine, norepinephrine ____

17. Which of the following is *not* part of the body's stress response?
    a. blood pressure rises   c. kidneys release fluids
    b. digestion stops   d. muscle tone increases   ____

18. Prolonged adrenaline secretion can cause which of the following?
    a. atherosclerosis   c. fever
    b. depression   d. ischemia   ____

19. The body's primary sensations include all of the following *except*:
    a. heat
    c. taste
    b. pain
    d. touch _____

20. Pain is the result of stimulation to specialized nerve ends called:
    a. inflictors
    c. receptors
    b. noceoceptors
    d. viscera _____

21. _____ has a primarily protective function in that it warns of tissue damage or destruction somewhere in the body.
    a. Adrenaline
    c. Pain
    b. Atherosclerosis
    d. Stress _____

22. Noceoceptors are found in all of the following *except* the:
    a. arterial walls
    c. muscles
    b. joints
    d. periosteum of the bones _____

23. Which of the following is a psychological response to pain?
    a. intensified alertness
    c. increased blood pressure
    b. blood flow to muscles
    d. anxiety _____

24. A syndrome of interest to the massage therapist is the _____ cycle associated with muscle spasms.
    a. pain-spasm-pain
    c. stress-spasm
    b. ischemic-pain
    d. reflex-reaction _____

25. _____ is localized tissue anemia due to obstruction of blood inflow.
    a. Infection
    c. Ischemia
    b. Inflammation
    d. Muscle spasm _____

26. All of the following are disease-producing microorganisms *except*:
    a. bacteria
    c. infections
    b. fungi
    d. viruses _____

27. When invading organisms are confined to a small area of the body, a _____ infection results.
    a. fungal
    c. parasitic
    b. local
    d. systemic _____

28. _____, minute, unicellular organisms with both plant and animal characteristics, are classified as harmless or harmful.
    a. Viruses
    c. Fungi
    b. Bacteria
    d. Parasites _____

29. When tissue is damaged, substances are released that cause dramatic secondary reactions collectively called:
    a. inflammation
    c. ischemia
    b. fever
    d. irritation
    ____

30. All of the following are signs of inflammation *except*:
    a. heat
    c. paleness
    b. swelling
    d. pain
    ____

31. In a process called _____, increased numbers of white blood cells engulf and digest invading organisms.
    a. leukocyte
    c. inflammation
    b. phagocytosis
    d. infection
    ____

32. Fever above 102 degrees F is classified as:
    a. prolonged
    c. high
    b. extreme
    d. early
    ____

33. When a client has a fever, massage is:
    a. restful
    c. gentle
    b. contraindicated
    d. supportive
    ____

34. Which of the following repair with noticeable scarring and weakness?
    a. bones and ligaments
    c. neurons
    b. muscles and tendons
    d. surface tissues
    ____

35. Which of the following repair slowly and may require immobilization?
    a. bones and ligaments
    c. neurons
    b. muscles and tendons
    d. surface tissues
    ____

36. Connective tissue cells called _____ provide structure for regenerating vascular and epithelial tissue.
    a. adhesions
    c. fibroblasts
    b. scar tissues
    d. neurons
    ____

37. Dense fibrous tissue that forms as an injury, a wound, a burn, or a sore heals is a:
    a. fibroblast
    c. neuron
    b. scar
    d. no answers
    ____

38. _____ is a set of behaviors and habits that positively influence health.
    a. Reflexism
    b. Optimism
    c. Physicality
    d. Wellness
    ____

39. On a wellness scale, "0" indicates:
    a. no perceivable sickness
    b. optimum health
    c. poor attitude
    d. severe illness
    ____

40. In medical terminology, a suffix often denotes a:
    a. diagnosis
    b. location
    c. relation
    d. structure
    ____

41. In medical terms, the prefix that means *half* is:
    a. epi-
    b. hemi-
    c. supra-
    d. uni-
    ____

42. When used in a medical term, the suffix -cyte means which of the following?
    a. condition
    b. disease
    c. tumor
    d. cell
    ____

43. When used in a medical term, which of the following stems means *rib*?
    a. ven
    b. throm
    c. hist
    d. cost
    ____

Part 2: Human Anatomy and Physiology

CHAPTER 5 —HUMAN ANATOMY AND PHYSIOLOGY

MULTIPLE CHOICE

1. The study of disease and disease processes is called:
   a. morphology
   b. physiology
   c. pathology
   d. anatomy ____

2. The scientific study of muscular activity and the mechanics of body movement is called:
   a. pathology
   b. morphology
   c. physiology
   d. kinesiology ____

3. Cells are organized into layers or groups called:
   a. tissues
   b. organs
   c. membranes
   d. atoms ____

4. Organ systems are arranged to form a(n):
   a. cell
   b. tissue
   c. membrane
   d. organism ____

5. Collections of similar cells that carry out specific bodily functions are called:
   a. centrosomes
   b. tissues
   c. organelles
   d. organs ____

6. In living cells, the central body or _____ contains the genetic information for continuing life.
   a. nucleus
   b. protoplasm
   c. cell membrane
   d. cytoplasm ____

7. During which stage of mitosis do chromosomes enlarge and become more defined?
   a. interphase
   b. telophase
   c. prophase
   d. anaphase ____

8. Most cellular work and growth are done during which stage of mitosis?
   a. interphase
   b. telophase
   c. prophase
   d. anaphase ____

9. In animals, the kind of cell division that occurs only in the sex glands and produces the egg and sperm needed for reproduction is:
   a. mitosis
   c. cytokinesis
   b. differentiation
   d. meiosis
   _____

10. The centriole and nucleus play an important role in which category of cell activity?
    a. vegetative
    c. specialized
    b. growth
    d. all answers
    _____

11. The two phases of metabolism are _____ and
    _____.
    a. mitosis, meiosis
    c. differentiation, mitosis
    b. anabolism, catabolism
    d. prophase, anaphase
    _____

12. Proteins that act as catalysts for chemical reactions in metabolism while remaining unchanged themselves are called:
    a. enzymes
    c. carbohydrates
    b. organelles
    d. tissues
    _____

13. The middle layer of cells in the zygote is the:
    a. endoderm
    c. ectoderm
    b. mesoderm
    d. dermis
    _____

14. Which of the following shape classifications of epithelial cells is flat?
    a. cuboidal
    c. stratified
    b. columnar
    d. squamous
    _____

15. The fibrous membrane that protects bone and serves as an attachment of tendons and ligaments is the:
    a. serous membrane
    c. skeletal membrane
    b. periosteum
    d. perichondrium
    _____

16. Cavities and capsules in and around joints are lined with a connective tissue membrane called the _____ membrane.
    a. synovial
    c. skeletal
    b. mucous
    d. periosteum
    _____

17. _____ tissue is loose connective tissue that binds the skin to underlying tissues and fills the spaces between muscles.
    a. Adipose
    c. Muscle
    b. Areolar
    d. Striated
    _____

18. Which type of muscle tissue is found in the hollow organs of the stomach, small intestine, colon, bladder, and the blood vessels?
    a. striated
    c. skeletal
    b. smooth
    d. cardiac
    _____

19. Skeletal muscles that can be activated by conscious effort are:
    a. voluntary
    c. adipose
    b. smooth
    d. cardiac
    _____

20. Which type of loose connective tissue provides the framework of the liver and other lymphoid organs?
    a. adipose
    c. hyaline
    b. areolar
    d. reticular
    _____

21. The white, glistening cords or bands that attach muscle to bone and consist mostly of tough collagen fibers are called:
    a. ligaments
    c. tendons
    b. adiposes
    d. fascia
    _____

22. _____ cartilage, the most resilient, is found in the external ear, larynx, and like structures.
    a. Fibrous
    c. Elastic
    b. Hyaline
    d. Embedded
    _____

23. Connective tissue represented by blood and lymph is called _____ tissue.
    a. smooth
    c. deep
    b. liquid
    d. cartilage
    _____

24. The _____ plane is an imaginary line that divides the body horizontally into upper and lower portions.
    a. coronal
    c. transverse
    b. sagittal
    d. midsagittal
    _____

25. Caudal or inferior aspect means situated toward the:
    a. midline
    c. left side
    b. crown of the head
    d. feet
    _____

26. Which of the following is a ventral cavity?
    a. abdominal
    c. thoracic
    b. pelvic
    d. all answers
    _____

27. The name for the region of the abdomen lateral to the epigastric region is:
    a. hypochondrium
    c. umbilical
    b. hypogastric
    d. inguinal
    _____

28. All of the following are part of the integumentary system except the:
    a. skin
    b. nails
    c. blood
    d. hair
    _____

29. Which skin layer contains fat cells, blood and lymph vessels, sweat and oil glands, hair follicles, and nerve endings?
    a. papillary
    b. epidermis
    c. reticular
    d. melanin
    _____

30. Hair and nails are composed of _____, a protein found in different form in skin.
    a. collagen
    b. hard keratin
    c. melanin
    d. elastin
    _____

31. A primary skin lesion that is a solid lump larger than a papule is a:
    a. fissure
    b. wheal
    c. tubercle
    d. macule
    _____

32. A superficial, thickened patch of epidermis caused by friction on the hands and feet is a(n):
    a. asteatosis
    b. keratoma
    c. steatoma
    d. impetigo
    _____

33. The most serious but least common skin cancer is:
    a. basal cell carcinoma
    b. squamous cell carcinoma
    c. malignant melanoma
    d. lymphatic cell carcinoma
    _____

34. The acute inflammation of a nerve trunk by the herpes varicella-zoster virus is:
    a. shingles
    b. Herpes simplex Type I
    c. Herpes simplex Type II
    d. Herpes Whitlow
    _____

35. Which of the following is characterized by red, raised lesions accompanied by the severe itching of an allergic reaction?
    a. contact dermatitis
    b. urticaria
    c. psoriasis
    d. eczema
    _____

36. A lentigine is also called a:
    a. birthmark
    b. liver spot
    c. freckle
    d. moth patch
    _____

37. Vertebrae are an example of which type of bone?
    a. long
    b. short
    c. flat
    d. irregular
    _____

38. The connective tissue filling the cavities of bones is called:
    a. compact bone tissue   c. spongy bone
    b. marrow   d. hyaline   ____

39. Which of the following supports the base of the tongue?
    a. cranium   c. maxilla
    b. hyoid bone   d. carpals   ____

40. Which type of joint has limited motion?
    a. synarthrotic   c. amphiarthrotic
    b. diarthrotic   d. synovial   ____

41. Which type of cartilage has a high density of collagen fibers and
    forms amphiarthrotic, cartilaginous joints?
    a. fibro   c. elastic
    b. hyaline   d. synovial   ____

42. _____ joints move through one plane, such as in the
    elbow.
    a. Hinge   c. Saddle
    b. Pivot   d. Gliding   ____

43. A _____ occurs when a bone is displaced in a joint.
    a. sprain   c. herniated disk
    b. dislocation   d. fracture   ____

44. _____ is a lateral curvature of the spine that involves
    vertebra rotation.
    a. Lordosis   c. Scoliosis
    b. Kyphosis   d. Scheuermann's kyphosis   ____

45. Which type of muscle does not attach to bone but can maintain a
    contraction for a long time without fatiguing easily?
    a. skeletal   c. voluntary
    b. smooth   d. striated   ____

46. The ability of muscle to stretch is called:
    a. irritability   c. elasticity
    b. contractility   d. extensibility   ____

47. Fascia project beyond muscle ends to become flat, tendonous
    sheaths called _____, which connect muscles to other
    structures.
    a. aponeuroses   c. fascicles
    b. ligaments   d. perimysium   ____

48. The term _____ refers to the combination of muscle tissue and its related connective tissue or fascia.
    a. endomysium
    b. perimysium
    c. myofascial
    d. fascicle

    ____

49. The cell wall of the muscle cell is the:
    a. myofibril
    b. sarcolemma
    c. sarcomere
    d. myosin

    ____

50. The channels in muscle cells, which have extracellular fluid that helps transmit nerve impulses through the cells, are the:
    a. transverse tubules
    b. sarcoplasmic reticula
    c. sarcolemma
    d. myoneural junctions

    ____

51. Which of the following, found in the belly of muscle, alerts the central nervous system to muscle length, stretch, and speed?
    a. actin
    b. spindle cells
    c. myosin
    d. myoneural junctions

    ____

52. The process in which glucose is broken down in the absence of oxygen is _____ respiration.
    a. aerobic
    b. anaerobic
    c. aerobic and anaerobic
    d. neither aerobic nor anaerobic

    ____

53. Which type of muscle fibers are found in large quantities in postural muscles?
    a. I
    b. II
    c. IIa
    d. IIb

    ____

54. Which of the following are not phasic muscles?
    a. gluteals
    b. rhomboids
    c. hamstrings
    d. gastrocnemiuses

    ____

55. Muscles that stabilize body parts so other muscles can act on adjacent limbs or body parts are called:
    a. synergists
    b. agonists
    c. fixators
    d. prime movers

    ____

56. Which of the following terms means "situated lower"?
    a. dorsal
    b. posterior
    c. distal
    d. inferior

    ____

57. When they alternate between contraction and relaxation, muscle spasms are called:
   a. tonic
   b. clonic
   c. chronic
   d. spasmodic
   _____

58. Which of the following muscles flexes, laterally rotates, and abducts the thigh?
   a. dorsal interosseus
   b. sartorius
   c. popliteus
   d. semispinalis
   _____

59. Which of the following is the main muscle of respiration?
   a. quadratus limborum
   b. diaphragm
   c. sternohyoid
   d. buccinator
   _____

60. The cardiac muscle is the:
   a. endocardium
   b. myocardium
   c. pericardium
   d. no answers
   _____

61. The _____ valve of the heart allows blood to pump from the left ventricle into the aorta.
   a. bicuspid
   b. mitral
   c. aortic semilunar
   d. pulmonary semilunar
   _____

62. In a normal adult, the heart beats about _____ to _____ times per minute.
   a. 50, 60
   b. 60, 80
   c. 80, 100
   d. 100, 120
   _____

63. Thick-walled muscular and elastic vessels that transport oxygenated blood from the heart are called:
   a. arterioles
   b. capillaries
   c. venules
   d. arteries
   _____

64. The main artery of the body is the:
   a. capillary
   b. vein
   c. aorta
   d. arteriole
   _____

65. The process by which blood pressure pushes fluids and substances through the capillary wall and into the tissue spaces is:
   a. filtration
   b. diffusion
   c. vasodilation
   d. vasoconstriction
   _____

66. In the phenomenon known as _____, muscles contract and exert external pressure on veins, tending to collapse them.
   a. diffusion
   b. venous pump
   c. filtration
   d. no answers
   _____

67. Blood circulation from the heart to the lungs and back to the heart is _____ circulation.
   a. general
   b. pulmonary
   c. systemic
   d. cardiac   ____

68. Which of the following increases the likelihood of atherosclerosis?
   a. high blood pressure
   b. smoking
   c. high cholesterol level
   d. all answers   ____

69. A cerebrovascular accident (CVA) or stroke is caused by a disturbance in cerebral circulation due to all of the following *except*:
   a. embolism
   b. atherosclerosis
   c. edema
   d. hemorrhage   ____

70. *Myocardial infarction* is another name for which of the following?
   a. heart attack
   b. blood clot
   c. aneurysm
   d. stroke   ____

71. The condition of excess fluid in the interstitial spaces is:
   a. hematoma
   b. edema
   c. angina pectoris
   d. stroke   ____

72. The skin may hold as much as _____ of all the body's blood.
   a. one-fourth
   b. one-third
   c. one-half
   d. two-thirds   ____

73. The iron-protein compound in red blood cells capable of carrying oxygen from the lungs to the cells and carbon dioxide from the cells is:
   a. hematoma
   b. erythrocyte
   c. leukocyte
   d. hemoglobin   ____

74. The process by which leukocytes engulf and digest harmful bacteria is:
   a. diffusion
   b. phagocytosis
   c. thrombocytosis
   d. coagulation   ____

75. In _____ anemia, which is inherited, hemoglobin molecules assume rodlike shapes after delivering oxygen to cells.
   a. aplastic
   b. sickle cell
   c. nutritional
   d. hemophilia   ____

76. Lymphatic capillaries located in the villi of the small intestine are called:
    a. lymphatics
    b. arterioles
    c. lacteals
    d. thoracic ducts
    _____

77. An inguinal lymph node is found where in the body?
    a. armpit
    b. breast
    c. elbow
    d. groin
    _____

78. Anything that can trigger an immune response is called a(n):
    a. antibody
    b. antigen
    c. leukocyte
    d. lymphocyte
    _____

79. B-cells work chiefly by producing:
    a. antigens
    b. allergens
    c. antibodies
    d. all answers
    _____

80. Blood cells that can engulf and digest cellular debris and foreign bodies in tissues are called:
    a. phagocytes
    b. leukocytes
    c. leukotrienes
    d. histamines
    _____

81. The junction where nerve signals jump from one nerve to another is called a:
    a. dendrite
    b. synapse
    c. neurotransmitter
    d. neuron
    _____

82. _____ neurons carry impulses from sense organs to the brain.
    a. Motor
    b. Sensory
    c. Efferent
    d. Internuncial
    _____

83. _____ is an acute inflammation of the pia mater and arachnoid mater around the brain and spinal cord.
    a. Encephalitis
    b. Diencephalitis
    c. Meningitis
    d. no answers
    _____

84. Which part of the brain helps maintain body balance, coordinate voluntary muscles, and smooth muscular movement?
    a. cerebrum
    b. cerebellum
    c. diencephalon
    d. brain stem
    _____

85. Which of the following cranial nerves controls tongue movement?
    a. hypoglossal
    b. abducent
    c. optic
    d. vagus
    _____

86. The _____ plexus consists of the four upper cervical nerves that supply the skin and control head, neck, and shoulder movement.
    a. sacral
    b. brachial
    c. cervical
    d. lumbar   ____

87. Which of the following is *not* an abdominal nerve?
    a. hypogastric
    b. lumar
    c. intercostal
    d. trigeminal   ____

88. The simplest form of nervous activity, which includes a sensory and motor nerve, is:
    a. kinesthesia
    b. reflex
    c. proprioception
    d. exteroception   ____

89. _____ sense where the body is and how it moves.
    a. Chemoreceptors
    b. Nociceptors
    c. Proprioceptors
    d. Exteroceptors   ____

90. Which of the following diseases results from breakdown of the myelin sheath?
    a. Parkinson's disease
    b. multiple sclerosis
    c. Parkinson's disease and multiple sclerosis
    d. neither Parkinson's disease nor multiple sclerosis   ____

91. Which of the following hormones is released by the pancreatic islets and helps transport glucose into cells?
    a. insulin
    b. calcitonin
    c. glucagon
    d. cortisol   ____

92. Which of the following pituitary hormones stimulates milk production in a woman's breast?
    a. adrenocorticotropic hormone
    b. prolactin
    c. gonadotropic hormone
    d. oxytocin   ____

93. A strained, tense facial expression and bulging eyes are characteristics of:
    a. Addison's disease
    b. goiter
    c. cretinism
    d. Graves' disease   ____

94. _____ is a sustained muscle contraction that usually affects the hands and feet.
    a. Goiter
    b. Tetany
    c. Cretinism
    d. Acromegaly   ____

95. _____, which results from excess glucocorticoid production, is characterized by obesity, muscle weakness, and elevated blood sugar.
    a. Addison's disease
    b. Cushing's syndrome
    c. Diabetes mellitus
    d. Graves' disease
    ____

96. The levels of respiration include all of the following *except*:
    a. cellular
    b. internal
    c. postural
    d. external
    ____

97. Which of the following helps keep the respiratory system functioning normally?
    a. regular exercise
    b. deep breathing
    c. healthy diet
    d. all answers
    ____

98. Which of the following begins as a bacterial infection that can incubate without detection by sealing itself in fleshy pockets?
    a. sinusitis
    b. pneumonia
    c. influenza
    d. tuberculosis
    ____

99. Which of the following is a main function of the digestive system?
    a. absorption
    b. digestion
    c. absorption and digestion
    d. neither absorption nor digestion
    ____

100. Which of the following is *not* a part of the alimentary canal?
    a. mouth
    b. esophagus
    c. liver
    d. stomach
    ____

101. Which of the following is part of the physical means of digestion?
    a. tongue
    b. pharynx msucles
    c. teeth
    d. all answers
    ____

102. Which layer of the alimentary canal is the outermost one?
    a. mucosa
    b. submucosa
    c. serous
    d. muscular
    ____

103. The mixture of digestive juices, mucus, and food material in the stomach is called:
    a. chyme
    b. bolus
    c. ileum
    d. mucosa
    ____

104. Bile from the liver and gallbladder is essential for the breakdown of:
   a. carbohydrates
   c. proteins
   b. fats
   d. all answers
   _____

105. Pepsin is found in which digestive juice?
   a. saliva
   c. pancreatic juice
   b. gastric juice
   d. bile
   _____

106. Which of the following is *not* found in pancreatic juice?
   a. trypsin
   c. lipase
   b. lactase
   d. amylase
   _____

107. Functions of the colon include all of the following *except*:
   a. excreting waste products
   c. producing bile
   b. storing waste products
   d. regulating water balance
   _____

108. When retained, metabolic wastes tend to:
   a. cause obesity
   c. poison the body
   b. ease bodily stress
   d. all answers
   _____

109. Which excretory organ eliminates water and heat through the process of perspiration?
   a. liver
   c. lungs
   b. kidneys
   d. skin
   _____

110. The bean-shaped glands that filter blood are called:
   a. nephrons
   c. ureters
   b. kidneys
   d. no answers
   _____

111. The kidneys have _____ to _____ nephrons.
   a. 2,000, 3,000
   c. 2 million, 3 million
   b. 50,000, 100,000
   d. 10 million, 15 million
   _____

112. Which of the following is *not* a function of the kidneys?
   a. maintain water balance
   c. balance acids and bases
   b. store glycogen
   d. produce renin
   _____

113. A sex gland that produces the reproductive cell is a(n):
   a. gonad
   c. ovum
   b. gamete
   d. zygote
   _____

114. The male reproductive system includes all of the following *except* the:
   a. vas deferens
   c. oviducts
   b. prostate gland
   d. Cowper's glands
   _____

115. The male gonads are outside the body in a pouch at the base of and below the penis called the:
   a. scrotum
   b. spermatid
   c. exocrine gland
   d. penis
   ____

116. Near the vestibule of the vagina are mucus-producing glands called the _____ glands.
   a. Bartholen's
   b. Cowper's
   c. endocrine
   d. no answers
   ____

117. The egg-carrying tubes of the female reproductive system are the:
   a. ovaries
   b. oviducts
   c. ovaries and oviducts
   d. neither ovaries nor oviducts
   ____

118. The glandular organs within the pelvic area are the:
   a. ovaries
   b. oviducts
   c. ovum
   d. vulva
   ____

119. The ovaries function to produce which of the following?
   a. ovum
   b. estrogen
   c. progesterone
   d. all answers
   ____

120. _____ is the hormone from the pituitary gland that transforms the follicle into the corpus *luteum*.
   a. Estrogen
   b. Luteinizing hormone
   c. Prolactin
   d. Testosterone
   ____

121. The physiological cessation of the menstrual cycle is called:
   a. maturation
   b. menstruation
   c. menopause
   d. gestation
   ____

122. Human gestation is normally how long?
   a. 300 days
   b. 40 weeks
   c. 200 days
   d. 25 weeks
   ____

123. From the beginning of the third month of pregnancy until birth, the developing child is called a(n):
   a. embryo
   b. gamete
   c. fetus
   d. zygote
   ____

Part 3: Massage Practice

CHAPTER 6 — EFFECTS, BENEFITS, INDICATIONS, AND CONTRAINDICATIONS OF MASSAGE

MULTIPLE CHOICE

1. _____ is a natural method by which minor aches and pains can be soothed while bringing tension and fatigue relief.
   a. Aneurosa
   b. Hematoma
   c. Massage
   d. Reflexology _____

2. Traditional Western massage is commonly also known as _____ massage.
   a. contraindicated
   b. natural
   c. petrissage
   d. Swedish _____

3. When a particular intervention or treatment is deemed detrimental or unsafe, that treatment is:
   a. effective
   b. referred
   c. contraindicated
   d. questionable _____

4. Physically, massage increases all of the following *except*:
   a. healing
   b. lymphatic function
   c. metabolism
   d. muscle spasms _____

5. Massage therapy effectively manages pain for all of the following conditions *except*:
   a. arthritis
   b. impetigo
   c. neuralgia
   d. sciatica _____

6. The direct physical effects of massage techniques on the tissues they contact are called _____ effects.
   a. contraindicated
   b. indirect
   c. mechanical
   d. reflex _____

7. The skin reddens or warms due to:
   a. increased sebaceous gland activity
   c. decreased sudoriferous gland activity
   b. increased lymph flow
   d. heightened blood circulation _____

8. The _____ gland is also called the sweat gland.
   a. adrenal
   c. sebaceous
   b. pituitary
   d. sudoriferous _____

9. _____ effects of massage are indirect responses to touch that affect body function through the nervous or energy systems.
   a. Mechanical
   c. Reflex
   b. Nutritional
   d. Trigger _____

10. Which of the following is a reflex effect of massage on the muscular system?
    a. compressed connective tissues
    c. stretched connective tissues
    b. hyperemia
    d. enhanced circulation _____

11. Massage can release fascial restrictions and reduce the thickening of connective tissues called:
    a. hematoma
    c. hyperplasia
    b. homeostasis
    d. hyperthermia _____

12. All of the following are effects of passive massage movements *except*:
    a. lubricated joints
    c. relaxed muscles
    b. nourished skin
    d. strengthened muscles _____

13. _____ joint movements are exercises in which the voluntary muscles are contracted by the client and resisted or assisted by the therapist.
    a. Active
    c. Passive
    b. Mechanical
    d. Reflex _____

14. The _____ nervous system consists of the brain and spinal cord.
    a. autonomic
    c. peripheral
    b. central
    d. parasympathetic _____

15. The sympathetic nervous system and the parasympathetic nervous system compose the _____ nervous system.
    a. autonomic
    c. peripheral
    b. central
    d. sympathetic _____

16. The _____ nervous system functions to conserve energy and reverse the action of the sympathetic division.
    a. autonomic
    c. parasympathetic
    b. central
    d. peripheral _____

17. The _____ nervous system consists of all the nerves that connect the central nervous system to the rest of the body.
    a. autonomic
    c. peripheral
    b. parasympathetic
    d. sympathetic
    _____

18. Sedative massage techniques include all of the following *except*:
    a. gentle stroking
    c. petrissage
    b. light friction
    d. vibration
    _____

19. Which of the following is *not* a stimulating massage technique?
    a. percussion
    c. rolling
    b. petrissage
    d. wringing
    _____

20. The _____ nervous system prepares the body to expend energy in response to emergencies, often called "fight-or-flight" preparation.
    a. autonomic
    c. peripheral
    b. parasympathetic
    d. sympathetic
    _____

21. Stimulation of the sympathetic nervous system results in all of the following *except*:
    a. accelerated heart rate
    c. decreased adrenal secretions
    b. activated sweat glands
    d. inhibited digestion
    _____

22. The body's internal balance is called:
    a. hematoma
    c. ischemia
    b. homeostasis
    d. restoration
    _____

23. The _____ and _____ nervous systems work together to maintain homeostasis.
    a. sympathetic, parasympathetic
    c. central, peripheral
    b. autonomic, central
    d. central, sympathetic
    _____

24. Massage increases levels of all of the following *except*:
    a. dopamine
    c. norepinephrine
    b. enkephalin
    d. serotonin
    _____

25. _____ is the "fight or flight" hormone that is active in the brain.
    a. Dopamine
    c. Norepinephrine
    b. Epinephrine
    d. Serotonin
    _____

26. A decline of _____ in the brain is linked to cognitive and
    movement problems.
    a. adrenaline   c. epinephrine
    b. dopamine   d. serotonin   _____

27. _____ is a neurotransmitter that promotes a sense of calm
    and well-being.
    a. Dopamine   c. Norepinephrine
    b. Epinephrine   d. Serotonin   _____

28. _____ and _____ are related to feelings of
    euphoria, appetite control, and enhancement of the immune
    system.
    a. Adrenaline, dopamine   c. Epinephrine,
                                            norepinephrine
    b. Enkephalins, endorphins   d. Serotonin, dopamine   _____

29. According to _____ theory, the positive effects of relaxing
    massage interrupt the transmission of pain sensations.
    a. endorphin   c. gate control
    b. pain control   d. homeostasis   _____

30. Which of the following is an effect of massage on the circulatory
    system?
    a. increased red blood cells   c. increased heart rate
    b. decreased cellular nutrition   d. greater adrenal secretions   _____

31. Swedish massage movements are always toward the:
    a. feet   c. heart
    b. head   d. lymph   _____

32. Which massage technique results in an almost instantaneous,
    though temporary, dilation of the capillaries?
    a. deep stroking   c. light stroking
    b. friction   d. percussion   _____

33. _____ hastens blood flow through the superficial veins,
    increases capillary-bed permeability, and increases the flow of
    interstitial fluid.
    a. Compression   c. Friction
    b. Deep stroking   d. Petrissage   _____

34. All of the following conditions are frequently relieved by regular
    massage treatment *except*:
    a. headache   c. joint pain
    b. intoxication   d. shoulder pain   _____

35. _____ contraindications require therapists to adjust massage for health concerns or to avoid discomfort or adverse effects.
    a. Conditional
    b. Regional
    c. Absolute
    d. Partial _____

36. Most massage contraindications are:
    a. absolute
    b. conditional
    c. partial
    d. regional _____

37. Which of the following is *not* a major contraindication for massage?
    a. inflammation
    b. abnormal body temperature
    c. cancer
    d. acute infectious disease _____

38. All of the following are signs of inflammation *except*:
    a. heat
    b. swelling
    c. pain
    d. hematoma _____

39. _____ is a condition that leads to bone deterioration.
    a. Inflammation
    b. Osteoporosis
    c. Edema
    d. Phlebitis _____

40. Which of the following best defines the term *phlebitis*?
    a. inflammation of veins due to blood clots
    b. blood clots loose and floating in blood
    c. vein inflammation accompanied by pain and swelling
    d. local artery distention due to a weakened wall _____

41. Another term for *bruise* is:
    a. aneurysm
    b. contusion
    c. edema
    d. scar _____

42. Which of the following can result from an imbalance of the factors regulating the interchange of fluids between capillaries and tissue spaces?
    a. contusion
    b. edema
    c. hematoma
    d. phlebitis _____

43. The congenital or genetic condition in which part of the lymphatic system develops incompletely is called:
    a. generalized malaise
    b. primary lymphedema
    c. secondary lymphedema
    d. Vodder's disease _____

44. _____ is the uncontrolled growth and spread of abnormal cells in the body.
    a. Aneurosa
    b. Cancer
    c. Edema
    d. Inflammation
    ____

45. Intoxication is contraindicated for massage because:
    a. lymph flow is restricted
    b. all acute inflammations are contraindicated
    c. intoxication causes edema
    d. massage can spread toxins and overstress the liver
    ____

46. During the second and third trimesters of pregnancy, which massage position is contraindicated?
    a. prone
    b. seated
    c. semi-reclining
    d. side-lying
    ____

47. All of the following are skin conditions contraindicated for massage *except*:
    a. acne
    b. skin tags
    c. warts
    d. edema
    ____

48. Which endangerment site is located at the posterior aspect of the knee?
    a. medial bracheum
    b. popliteal fossa
    c. axilla
    d. femoral triangle
    ____

49. _____ warrant consideration when being massaged due to their delicate, relatively unprotected underlying anatomical structures.
    a. Pressure sites
    b. Manipulative areas
    c. Endangerment sites
    d. Distress locations
    ____

Part 3: Massage Practice

CHAPTER 7—EQUIPMENT AND PRODUCTS

MULTIPLE CHOICE

1. All of the following are ways in which massage practitioners demonstrate professionalism *except*:
   a. appearance
   b. financial statements
   c. good manners
   d. speech _____

2. When considering client comfort, which of the following is *not* important?
   a. ventilation
   b. adequate heat
   c. indirect lighting
   d. furnishings _____

3. A 1990 survey indicated that about _____ of massage therapists practice in health clubs, resorts, or spas.
   a. one-fourth
   b. one-third
   c. one-half
   d. two-thirds _____

4. According to a 2007 Federation of Massage Therapy Boards survey, _____ percent of therapists work from home.
   a. 15
   b. 20
   c. 40
   d. 60 _____

5. Whatever the location of the massage facility, standards of cleanliness, safety, and _____ must be observed.
   a. professionalism
   b. relaxation
   c. order
   d. marketing _____

6. Clients entering a massage business will be influenced by the environment and:
   a. location
   b. lighting
   c. people
   d. no answers _____

7. In a massage practice, the main concern is protection of the client's:
   a. health and comfort
   b. relaxation
   c. massage interest
   d. time and money _____

8. Which of the following is *not* considered one of the three areas of operation or activity in a massage business?
   a. business
   b. hydrotherapy
   c. massage
   d. storage

   _____

9. In a massage business, client consultations are usually done in the _____ area.
   a. hydrotherapy
   b. bathroom
   c. massage
   d. business

   _____

10. Because massage tends to stimulate _____, every massage area must have access to a clean restroom.
    a. blood pressure
    b. kidney activity
    c. oil secretion
    d. blood circulation

    _____

11. In a typical massage business, which of the following is found in the massage area?
    a. analgesic oil
    b. appointment book
    c. business telephone
    d. shampoo

    _____

12. In a massage business, which of the following is *not* kept in the business area?
    a. bolster
    b. filing system
    c. stationery
    d. telephone

    _____

13. In a massage business, the _____ must be at least 10 feet wide and 12 feet long.
    a. business area
    b. bathroom
    c. massage room
    d. storage room

    _____

14. The massage practitioner can sit while working on all of the following *except* the client's:
    a. back
    b. face
    c. feet
    d. hands

    _____

15. In the massage area, a temperature of _____ degrees F is considered too warm.
    a. 65
    b. 72
    c. 75
    d. 78

    _____

16. In a massage room that is cooler than preferred, which of the following should be used to ensure the client's warmth?
    a. body heat
    b. candles
    c. cool cloths
    d. electric mattress pads

    _____

17. For proper relaxation, the client needs a good supply of:
    a. fresh air
    b. coffee
    c. linens
    d. no answers
    _____

18. In the massage area, the preferred lighting is:
    a. direct
    b. reflective
    c. glaring
    d. blue
    _____

19. Soothing music can be used to mask which of the following in the massage area?
    a. overheating
    b. painful techniques
    c. harsh lighting
    d. outside noise
    _____

20. In the massage area, client and practitioner comfort depend on the practitioner's massage table and:
    a. hands
    b. music
    c. stool
    d. temperature
    _____

21. Which of the following is a sign of a poorly constructed massage table?
    a. squeaking
    b. shaking
    c. rocking
    d. all answers
    _____

22. Which of the following is *not* a factor in determining the optimum height of a massage table?
    a. client size
    b. table weight
    c. massage style
    d. practitioner height
    _____

23. To measure massage table height, stand in an erect yet relaxed manner and measure the distance from the floor to the:
    a. center of the thigh
    b. tips of the fingers
    c. middle of the palm
    d. point of the waist
    _____

24. Pain in all of the following indicate that the massage table is too high for the practitioner *except* pain in the:
    a. arm
    b. lower back
    c. shoulder
    d. upper back
    _____

25. The optimal width of a massage table, including an additional inch of padding, is _____ inches.
    a. 27
    b. 28
    c. 29
    d. 30
    _____

26. A massage table wider than _____ inches may be awkward to use.
    a. 27
    b. 28
    c. 29
    d. 30
    _____

27. A massage table that is _____ inches long is optimal for tall clients.
   a. 68
   b. 70
   c. 72
   d. 76
   ____

28. Good-quality _____ is the best covering for a massage table because it is durable and easy to keep clean.
   a. leather
   b. cotton
   c. vinyl
   d. plastic
   ____

29. All of the following substances cause vinyl to become brittle and crack *except*:
   a. alcohol
   b. body oil
   c. chlorine bleach
   d. mild detergent
   ____

30. Accommodations for the face allow the client to lie face down with the cervical spine straight, taking strain off the:
   a. neck and lower back
   b. neck and upper back
   c. head and chest
   d. lower back and legs
   ____

31. Which of the following is *not* a feature to consider when buying a massage table?
   a. bolsters
   b. carrying case
   c. face rest
   d. warranty
   ____

32. When the massage client is face down, bolsters be placed under the _____ to reduce lower back strain.
   a. thighs
   b. head
   c. ankles
   d. knees
   ____

33. When laundry is done daily for the massage practice, there should be enough linens to last:
   a. one day
   b. two days
   c. one week
   d. one and a half weeks
   ____

34. Popular fabrics for massage practice sheets include all of the following *except*:
   a. cotton
   b. flannel
   c. percale
   d. vinyl
   ____

35. The most popular massage lubricants are oils and:
   a. creams
   b. lotions
   c. powders
   d. tinctures
   ____

36. Rancid massage oils are problematic because they:
    a. dry the skin   c. have an offensive odor
    b. provide natural nutrients   d. cause allergies   ____

37. Which of the following is a petroleum-based product *not*
    recommended for massage?
    a. olive oil   c. mineral oil
    b. sesame oil   d. cornstarch   ____

38. A drawback to using massage creams is:
    a. client allergies   c. offensive odor
    b. high cost   d. extreme oily quality   ____

39. Why might the massage practitioner prefer to buy massage
    lubricants in bulk?
    a. more economical   c. less likely to go rancid
    b. easier to store   d. better shipping rates   ____

40. What causes massage oil to become rancid?
    a. pressure   c. air
    b. lemon juice   d. essential oil   ____

41. Cornstarch may be preferable for clients with:
    a. dry skin   c. scent allergies
    b. oily skin   d. poor circulation   ____

42. What precaution must be taken when using powders as massage
    lubricants?
    a. avoid direct contact with skin c. do use on oily skin
    b. avoid inhaling   d. use in small quantities ____

43. When performing a patch test, a small amount of the product
    being tested is applied to the client's:
    a. cheek   c. forearm
    b. inner elbow   d. lower back   ____

44. All of the following indicate a reaction to a patch test *except*:
    a. itching   c. oiliness
    b. inflammation   d. stinging   ____

45. Which of the following can be used to remove excess oil from the
    client's skin following massage?
    a. alcohol   c. cornstarch
    b. antibacterial soap   d. mild detergent   ____

Part 3: Massage Practice

CHAPTER 8—SANITARY AND SAFETY PRACTICES

MULTIPLE CHOICE

1. Every state has laws that make the practice of _____ mandatory for the protection of public health.
   a. medicine
   b. business
   c. sanitation
   d. massage   ____

2. The nature of the _____ determines the extent of sanitation and sterilization procedures.
   a. business
   b. client
   c. facility
   d. practitioner   ____

3. The primary sanitation concern for the massage practitioner is that:
   a. clients who are contagious not be treated
   b. any item that contacts the client is clean and sanitary
   c. the practitioner has the skills needed to provide full-body massages
   d. the client and practitioner agree on all sanitary procedures   ____

4. The practitioner's hands must be sanitized by washing with soap and warm water:
   a. at the end of each session
   b. at the start of the work day
   c. at the end of the work day
   d. before touching each client   ____

5. All of the following are causes or sources of disease *except*:
   a. cancer
   b. genetics
   c. infectious agents
   d. lymph flow   ____

6. Disease-causing pathogens may be transmitted from an infected host to a new host:
   a. directly
   b. indirectly
   c. directly or indirectly
   d. neither directly nor indirectly   ____

7. To infect a new host, a pathogen must make contact with or _____ an organism, and then find entry.
   a. confront
   b. contaminate
   c. reproduce
   d. sterilize   ____

8. Which of the following is *not* a common path of infection?
   a. skin contact
   b. skin invasion
   c. virus
   d. ingestion _____

9. Pathogens enter the body in varied ways that can be called paths of:
   a. arrival
   b. manifestation
   c. reproduction
   d. transmission _____

10. All of the following are illnesses caused by organisms or parasites in contaminated food *except*:
    a. giardia
    b. hepatitis
    c. HIV
    d. typhoid _____

11. Tiny, airborne pathogens may be inhaled through close contact with a contagious individual who is:
    a. coughing
    b. sneezing
    c. talking
    d. all answers _____

12. Which of the following sexually transmitted diseases is contracted by direct contact with infected tissue?
    a. syphilis
    b. HIV
    c. gonorrhea
    d. herpes _____

13. What is the body's major defense against pathogen invasion?
    a. sterile gloves
    b. healthy, intact skin
    c. isolation technique
    d. antigens _____

14. When the surface of the skin is broken, the possibility of _____ increases drastically.
    a. respiratory infection
    b. pathogenic invasion
    c. food poisoning
    d. disinfection _____

15. Bacteria exist on the body in which of the following areas?
    a. skin
    b. under the nails
    c. body secretions
    d. all answers _____

16. Bacteria are numerous in all of the following *except*:
    a. dirt
    b. healthy body tissue
    c. refuse
    d. unclean water _____

17. *Germ* is another name for which pathogen?
    a. bacterium
    b. fungus
    c. parasite
    d. virus _____

18. Nonpathogenic bacteria are considered:
    a. beneficial   c. harmful
    b. disease producing   d. parasitic   ____

19. *Spirilla* is one of the three general forms of:
    a. bacteria   c. parasites
    b. fungi   d. viruses   ____

20. The living host of a parasite must be:
    a. animal   c. plant
    b. human   d. all answers   ____

21. Viruses invade living cells and control the cells' activity to produce:
    a. antigens   c. fungi
    b. bacteria   d. more viruses   ____

22. A virus may act as an antigen and cause the system to produce:
    a. HIV   c. bacteria
    b. antibodies   d. fungi   ____

23. _____, a diverse group of organisms potentially able to cause disease, thrive or grow in wet or damp areas.
    a. Bacteria   c. Parasites
    b. Fungi   d. Viruses   ____

24. Which of the following illnesses is caused by a fungus?
    a. AIDS   c. mumps
    b. candida   d. smallpox   ____

25. _____ is the body's natural ability to resist infection by harmful bacteria after they have entered the body.
    a. Pathogenesis   c. Inflammation
    b. Immunity   d. Leukocytosis   ____

26. The body produces _____, which inhibit or destroy harmful bacteria.
    a. antibodies   c. pathogens
    b. antigens   d. parasites   ____

27. Which of the following is *not* one of the three main levels of removing pathogens from implements and surfaces?
    a. disinfection   c. sanitation
    b. decontamination   d. sterilization   ____

28. Which process of pathogen removal is most time consuming?
   a. disinfection
   b. decontamination
   c. sanitation
   d. sterilization
   ____

29. Which process of pathogen removal is used to cleanse the hands?
   a. disinfection
   b. immunization
   c. sanitation
   d. sterilization
   ____

30. The massage practitioner's primary precaution in infection control is:
   a. sterilization
   b. contamination
   c. hand washing
   d. sanitation
   ____

31. Washing the hands after the massage protects the:
   a. client
   b. practitioner
   c. client and practitioner
   d. neither client nor practitioner
   ____

32. When there is concern that linens have been contaminated, _____ can be added to the wash water.
   a. cresol
   b. Lysol
   c. boric acid
   d. chlorine bleach
   ____

33. Which of the following is a general antiseptic?
   a. chlorine bleach
   b. hydrogen peroxide
   c. cresol
   d. Lysol
   ____

34. Which of the following is a disinfectant?
   a. water
   b. boric acid
   c. chlorine bleach
   d. soap and water
   ____

35. According to Universal Precautions, all blood and body fluids are to be considered potentially infectious for such diseases as:
   a. hepatitis A
   b. hepatitis C
   c. HIV
   d. all answers
   ____

36. A cover is provided for a wet sanitizer to prevent solution:
   a. contamination
   b. leakage
   c. decontamination
   d. sterilization
   ____

37. _____ is the method of boiling objects in water at 212 degrees F for about 20 minutes.
   a. Decontaminating
   b. Disinfecting
   c. Moist heating
   d. Wet sanitizing
   ____

38. A(n) _____ is sometimes used in the medical field for sterilization purposes.
    a. autoclave
    c. disinfectant
    b. cresol
    d. wet sanitizer
    _____

39. In the massage practice, surfaces, implements, and linens are disinfected using:
    a. boric acid
    c. moist heat
    b. chlorine bleach
    d. soap and water
    _____

40. Proper linen storage is a _____ safety consideration.
    a. client
    c. practitioner
    b. facility
    d. all answers
    _____

41. Which of the following is a recommended safety practice for fire safety?
    a. Store equipment and linens properly.
    b. Know the location of the first aid kit.
    c. Keep emergency information posted in plain view near all telephones.
    d. Be aware of evacuation procedures.
    _____

42. First aid is a safety consideration of the massage:
    a. client
    c. table
    b. facility
    d. practitioner
    _____

43. Which of the following is a safety precaution classified under practitioner personal safety?
    a. Know the location of the first aid kit.
    b. Maintain all equipment.
    c. Make sure all floors in wet areas are slip proof.
    d. Help clients on and off of the massage table.
    _____

Part 3: Massage Practice

CHAPTER 9—THE CONSULTATION

MULTIPLE CHOICE

1. Clients give pertinent information about who they are and why they are seeking the services of the therapist at:
   a. a preliminary consultation
   b. the beginning of the first massage session
   c. an open house
   d. the end of the first massage session ____

2. The extent of the consultation depends on the type of massage services offered and the:
   a. type of training the practitioner has
   b. reason the client has come for the session
   c. practitioner's hourly rate
   d. client's ability to pay for treatment ____

3. A relatively healthy client appearing for a wellness massage will require a(n):
   a. lengthy consultation
   b. doctor's referral
   c. brief consultation
   d. extensive training period ____

4. The purpose of screening prospective massage clients is to:
   a. save time for the practitioner
   b. eliminate inappropriate situations
   c. save time for the potential client
   d. all answers ____

5. Which of the following is *not* a question the massage practitioner should ask when screening potential clients?
   a. "How did you find out about my services?"
   b. "What is your experience with massage"
   c. "What is your main reason for making this appointment?"
   d. "How much are you able to pay for massage services?" ____

6. At a consultation, the practitioner should do all of the following *except*:
   a. state policies
   b. determine the practitioner's needs
   c. obtain informed consent
   d. explain procedures ____

7. The process that helps determine the course of treatment and sets the tone of the therapeutic relationship between therapist and client is the:
   a. consultation
   b. massage session
   c. SOAP session
   d. initial appointment   ____

8. Which of the following would *not* contribute to making a positive first impression?
   a. Be courteous and sensitive.
   b. Keep the consultation relaxed.
   c. Greet no clients formally.
   d. Be organized and ready.   ____

9. In an effective consultation, the practitioner:
   a. explains procedures
   b. listens to the client's needs
   c. explains policies
   d. all answers   ____

10. A good _____ provides the basis for trust, mutual respect, openness, and harmony, which enhance the therapeutic relationship.
    a. first impression
    b. rapport
    c. interview
    d. massage session   ____

11. All of the following personalize the client/practitioner connection *except*:
    a. maintaining visual contact
    b. listening attentively
    c. using the client's name
    d. mirroring the practitioner's language   ____

12. Nonverbal communication, sometimes known as _____, provides clues to a person's emotional or subconscious condition.
    a. body language
    b. verbal communication
    c. spoken language
    d. written language   ____

13. Posturing, gestures, and facial expressions are examples of:
    a. spoken language
    b. verbal expression
    c. nonverbal communication
    d. voice enhancements   ____

14. Which of the following may indicate the client is experiencing discomfort during a massage session?
    a. fidgeting
    b. flinches
    c. muscle contractions
    d. all answers   ____

15. Facial expressions like serene smiles and subtle sounds like moans provide _____ to the practitioner during the massage session.
    a. background noise
    b. feedback
    c. amusement
    d. warnings _____

16. Which of the following is positive body-language behavior for a practitioner who wants to appear open and interested?
    a. maintaining eye contact
    b. shuffling papers
    c. sitting behind a desk
    d. facing the back to the client _____

17. Which is the preferred question type for the practitioner during a client consultation?
    a. yes-or-no response
    b. multiple-choice
    c. explanatory response
    d. all answers _____

18. The preliminary consultation is the first opportunity for the client and therapist to:
    a. agree on some goals
    b. clarify their intentions
    c. meet one another
    d. all answers _____

19. Before providing informed consent, the client must receive information about the massage, including all of the following *except*:
    a. potential benefits of massage
    b. expectations for the massage
    c. names of other local massage practitioners
    d. possible undesirable effects of the massage _____

20. Massage practice policies should be presented in which format?
    a. posted on office walls
    b. printed on intake forms
    c. verbalized
    d. all answers _____

21. The practitioner's professional affiliations would be listed under which type of policy?
    a. business
    b. fee
    c. therapist qualifications
    d. services offered _____

22. All of the following are part of the policies for session procedures *except*:
    a. draping procedures
    b. therapy limitations
    c. massage sequence
    d. oil or lubricant use _____

23. Which of the following is a business policy for the massage practice?
    a. therapist's special training
    c. policies for sexual boundaries
    b. forms of payment accepted
    d. music use during sessions _____

24. What question should the massage practitioner ask to determine the client's expectation of and preference for massage?
    a. How did you find out about our massage services?
    b. Have you received massages before?
    c. Have you had any surgery?
    d. What do you do with the majority of your time? _____

25. Practitioners may ask clients how they found out about the massage practice to gain information about:
    a. potential health problems
    c. effective advertising
    b. clients' expectations
    d. stress-carrying areas _____

26. After a client indicates painful areas on a body diagram, the next step is to have the:
    a. client locate the areas on the body
    b. practitioner take notes on the diagram
    c. client add comments to the diagram
    d. practitioner describe the client's symptoms _____

27. A preliminary assessment includes a(n):
    a. client history
    c. observation
    b. examination
    d. all answers _____

28. Noticing how the client moves is part of which section of the preliminary assessment?
    a. examination
    c. intake
    b. history
    d. observation _____

29. Which part of the preliminary assessment includes descriptions offered by clients?
    a. examination
    c. intake
    b. history
    d. observation _____

30. A(n) _____ is an outline the practitioner can follow for several sessions when giving massage treatments.
    a. intake form
    c. client file
    b. general treatment strategy
    d. treatment plan _____

31. Which of the following provides past information about the client?
    a. intake form
    b. medical history form
    c. intake form and medical history form
    d. neither intake form nor medical history form _____

32. Which of the following ensures the client has received and understands the nature and extent of the massage services?
    a. treatment plan
    b. intake form
    c. client history
    d. informed consent _____

33. The client's right to modify or withdraw consent to continue treatment at any time during any session is:
    a. informed consent
    b. right to practice
    c. full right of refusal
    d. refusal of treatment _____

34. Which of the following statements about informed consent is most accurate?
    a. The practitioner may change procedures without renewing informed consent.
    b. Informed consent is an ongoing process.
    c. Verbal permission suffices for informed consent.
    d. Informed consent may never be retracted. _____

35. Information in a client file includes all of the following *except*:
    a. employment applications
    b. intake information
    c. SOAP notes
    d. treatment plan _____

36. All of the following are reasons for creating and maintaining client files *except*:
    a. providing quick access to client information
    b. providing a basis for creating treatment plans
    c. delivering legal evidence to reduce client liability
    d. exchanging client information with other health professionals _____

37. In the SOAP acronym of recording client and session information, the letter *S* stands for:
    a. sensory
    b. standard
    c. subconscious
    d. subjective _____

38. In which phase of the SOAP notes process are the therapist's treatment goals noted?
    a. assessment
    b. objective
    c. planning
    d. subjective _____

39. Information provided by the client about an aggravating condition is recorded in which phase of the SOAP notes process?
    a. assessment
    c. planning
    b. objective
    d. subjective ____

40. Recommendations suggested to the client are recorded in which phase of the SOAP notes procedure?
    a. assessment
    c. planning
    b. objective
    d. subjective ____

41. Reviewing updated records before a client arrives for a return visit can refresh the practitioner's memory about the:
    a. client's condition
    c. client's preferences
    b. treatments given
    d. all answers ____

42. Because the practitioner often works closely with a client's physician when dealing with certain physical conditions:
    a. information may be shared freely among practitioner, physician, and client
    b. the confidence of both client and physician must be respected
    c. the physician is required to disclose client information to the practitioner
    d. the practitioner is required to provide information to the physician ____

43. Massage practitioners who feel clients' physicians should be consulted before beginning massage treatments should:
    a. consult the physicians
    b. obtain written permission from the clients
    c. obtain verbal permission from the clients
    d. begin massage treatments ____

44. A release of information form contains all of the following *except*:
    a. client's name
    b. therapist's name
    c. name of the person information is being given to
    d. reason for release of information ____

45. Confidential client information may be shared without a signed release of information form when:
    a. ordered by a court of law
    b. requested by a physician
    c. requested by an insurance company
    d. deemed necessary by the therapist ____

Part 3: Massage Practice

CHAPTER 10—CLASSICAL MASSAGE MOVEMENTS

MULTIPLE CHOICE

1. Which of the following does *not* affect the delivery and outcome of massage?
   a. continuous interaction of client and therapist
   b. duration of the session
   c. intent with which each manipulation is delivered
   d. purpose of the session ____

2. The six major categories of Swedish massage include all of the following *except*:
   a. touch
   b. friction
   c. manipulation
   d. kneading ____

3. Which of the following categories of Swedish massage manipulations includes wringing?
   a. friction
   b. effleurage
   c. kneading movements
   d. joint movements ____

4. Which of the following is *not* a kneading movement in massage?
   a. fulling
   b. petrissage
   c. rolling
   d. skin rolling ____

5. Beating, slapping, and tapping are all examples of which type of massage movement?
   a. friction
   b. gliding
   c. percussion
   d. touch ____

6. Which of the following is a type of vibration massage movement?
   a. manual
   b. mechanical
   c. manual and mechanical
   d. neither manual nor mechanical ____

7. Which type of massage movement is categorized as passive or active?
   a. friction
   b. gliding
   c. joint movement
   d. kneading ____

8. Compression is an example of which type of massage movement?
   a. effleurage
   b. friction
   c. kneading
   d. percussion ____

9. Which of the following is a type of gliding movement?
   a. aura stroking   c. fulling
   b. compression   d. rolling   _____

10. Control of massage treatment results is possible when the practitioner regulates all of the following *except*:
    a. intensity of the pressure
    b. duration of each manipulation type
    c. speed of recovery
    d. speed, length, and direction of the movement   _____

11. Light massage movements are applied over:
    a. thin tissues or fleshy parts
    b. thin tissues or bony parts
    c. thick tissues or fleshy parts
    d. thick tissues or bony parts   _____

12. _____ movements are applied in a quick rhythm and are stimulating.
    a. Gentle   c. Light
    b. Heavy   d. Vigorous   _____

13. In Swedish massage, most manipulations are centripetal, or directed:
    a. away from the head   c. toward the head
    b. away from the heart   d. toward the heart   _____

14. Massage movements directed away from the heart are called:
    a. centrical   c. centripetal
    b. centrifugal   d. compression   _____

15. When a student is learning massage, a full-body massage takes about how long to perform?
    a. 30 minutes to 1 hour   c. $1\frac{1}{2}$ to 2 hours
    b. 1 hour   d. 3 hours   _____

16. The placing of the practitioner's hand, finger, or body part on the client without movement in any direction is called:
    a. compression   c. kneading
    b. friction   d. touch   _____

17. _____ refers to a number of massage strokes that manipulate one layer of soft tissue over or against another.
    a. Effleurage   c. Percussion
    b. Friction   d. Touch   _____

18. During a massage, what constitutes the first and last contact of the practitioner with the client?
    a. body language
    b. closure
    c. communication
    d. touch _____

19. What kind of touch give the client the chance to become more receptive to the practitioner's touch and presence?
    a. stationary contact
    b. noninvasive, superficial touch
    c. vibration
    d. percussion _____

20. All massage techniques use physical contact, but the quality and sense of touch convey the _____ and _____ of the movements.
    a. pressure, duration
    b. strength, meaning
    c. speed, length
    d. intent, power _____

21. Touch can be remarkably effective for:
    a. reducing pain
    b. lowering blood pressure
    c. controlling nervous irritability
    d. all answers _____

22. Deep pressure should be used when what type of effect is desired?
    a. anesthetizing
    b. calming
    c. stimulating
    d. all answers _____

23. To prevent self-injury when applying deep pressure, the massage practitioner should do which of the following?
    a. execute good body mechanics
    b. use only the heel of the hand
    c. apply deep pressure with compression
    d. use deep pressure sparingly _____

24. Which of the following gliding strokes requires very light pressure of the fingertips or hands with long, flowing strokes?
    a. aura stroking
    b. deep gliding
    c. feather stroking
    d. superficial gliding _____

25. Which massage movement is also called nerve stroking?
    a. aura stroking
    b. circular friction
    c. rolling
    d. feather stroking _____

26. The most frequently used manipulation in Swedish or Western massage is:
    a. effleurage
    b. friction
    c. kneading
    d. vibration _____

27. Which of the following is *not* a body part used by the practitioner to accomplish effleurage?
    a. knuckles
    b. palm of the hand
    c. back of the hand
    d. fingers
    _____

28. Over small areas like the face or hands, effleurage is performed with the:
    a. palm of the hand
    b. fingers or thumbs
    c. knuckles
    d. forearm
    _____

29. What massage movement is used to distribute lubricant?
    a. deep gliding
    b. compression
    c. superficial gliding
    d. fulling
    _____

30. Deep gliding strokes generally:
    a. follow the direction of muscle fibers
    b. flow toward the ends of the limbs
    c. are directed away from the center of the body
    d. are directed away from lymph flow
    _____

31. _____ is a manipulation uses enough pressure to have a mechanical effect.
    a. Compression
    b. Deep gliding
    c. Fulling
    d. Percussion
    _____

32. The effects and benefits of gliding massage strokes include all of the following *except*:
    a. cools tissue
    b. soothes tissue after deep work
    c. enhances lymph circulation
    d. prepares tissue for deep work
    _____

33. _____ is a kneading technique in which the practitioner tries to grasp tissue and gently lift and spread it.
    a. Chucking
    b. Fulling
    c. Rolling
    d. Skin rolling
    _____

34. The effects and benefits of petrissage include all of the following *except*:
    a. relaxes muscles
    b. improves cellular nutrition
    c. decreases metabolic wastes
    d. improves sensitivity to nerve impulses
    _____

35. _____ presses one layer of tissue against another layer to flatten, broaden, or stretch tissue.
   a. Compression
   b. Friction
   c. Effleurage
   d. Petrissage _____

36. Directional friction may be cross-fiber or:
   a. centripetal
   b. longitudinal
   c. circular
   d. superficial _____

37. The intention of _____ is to broaden, separate, and align fibrous tissue.
   a. compression
   b. cross-fiber friction
   c. circular friction
   d. kneading _____

38. Which massage movement is done with the whole hand (palm side) or the heel of the hand over large muscular areas?
   a. aura stroking
   b. fulling
   c. gliding
   d. palmar compression _____

39. The variations of friction used principally to massage the arms and legs include all of the following *except*:
   a. chucking
   b. rolling
   c. vibration
   d. wringing _____

40. In which friction movement do the hands stretch and twist flesh against bones in opposing directions?
   a. compression
   b. chucking
   c. rolling
   d. wringing _____

41. _____ allows for tension release by gently shaking a relaxed body part so that the flesh flops around the bone.
   a. Chucking
   b. Jostling
   c. Shaking
   d. Wringing _____

42. Which friction movement is most effective after muscles have exerted themselves, such as after a workout or competition?
   a. chucking
   b. jostling
   c. rocking
   d. wringing _____

43. Which friction movement is often used to desensitize a point or an area?
   a. rocking
   b. shaking
   c. vibration
   d. wringing _____

44. For which percussion movement does the practitioner use a softly clenched hand?
    a. beating
    b. cupping
    c. hacking
    d. tapping _____

45. Which percussion movement is very stimulating and uses rhythmical, glancing contact with the body?
    a. cupping
    b. hacking
    c. slapping
    d. tapping _____

46. _____ is a technique used by respiratory therapists to help break up lung congestion.
    a. Cupping
    b. Hacking
    c. Tapping
    d. Slapping _____

47. The percussion movement that is a rapid striking movement that can be done with the ulnar side of one or both hands is:
    a. beating
    b. hacking
    c. slapping
    d. tapping _____

48. Which classification of joint movement stretches the fibrous tissue and moves the joint through its range of motion?
    a. active
    b. active assistive
    c. active resistive
    d. passive _____

49. Which type of end feel is an abrupt restriction to a joint movement due to pain?
    a. soft
    b. hard
    c. empty
    d. springy _____

Part 3: Massage Practice

CHAPTER 11—APPLICATION OF MASSAGE TECHNIQUE

MULTIPLE CHOICE

1. In massage, which body part(s) provide(s) the practitioner's power?
   a. feet
   b. heart
   c. pelvis and torso
   d. arms and hands _____

2. In massage, the _____ provide communication with the client.
   a. pelvis and torso
   b. heart and lungs
   c. legs
   d. arms and hands _____

3. All of the following contribute to stress and can cause injury *except*:
   a. therapeutic massage
   b. improper posture
   c. poor body alignment
   d. sloppy technique _____

4. Practitioner burnout results when mental and emotional energy are not:
   a. increased
   b. replenished
   c. sustained
   d. all answers _____

5. Body mechanics are studied and incorporated to:
   a. conserve energy
   b. increase power
   c. reduce chances of injury
   d. all answers _____

6. Which of the following is important to maintain regular rhythm and control when doing slow or fast movements?
   a. hand flexibility
   b. hand mobility
   c. hand position
   d. hand size _____

7. Which of the following hand characteristics helps work the contours of the client's body and control speed and pressure?
   a. flexibility
   b. mobility
   c. size
   d. strength _____

8. The therapist must have well-trained hands and which of the following to move efficiently while applying varied massage movements?
   a. good sense of balance
   b. body control
   c. good sense of balance and body control
   d. neither good sense of balance nor body control ____

9. Body _____ is the observation of body postures relative to safe and efficient movement in daily living activities.
   a. strength
   b. mechanics
   c. weight
   d. mobility ____

10. A consistent forward posture of the head may cause what type of pain?
    a. upper back
    b. hand and wrist
    c. lower back
    d. neck and shoulder ____

11. To protect the hands, the practitioner should use what when applying pressure with the fingers or thumb?
    a. cushioned palmar side of thumb and fingers
    b. thumb only
    c. finger tips
    d. all answers ____

12. It is best to use the _____ and _____ to apply deep pressure.
    a. forearm, elbow
    b. fingers, palm
    c. hand, wrist
    d. hand, forearm ____

13. By keeping the hands relatively close to the center of the body, the knees slightly flexed, and the feet apart, the practitioner:
    a. aligns the back
    b. uses the arm muscles to deliver massage strokes
    c. uses the leg muscles to deliver massage strokes
    d. stresses the back ____

14. _____ is directly proportionate to the amount of stress and the amount of biomechanical deviation.
    a. Risk of injury
    b. Mobility
    c. Balance
    d. Posture ____

15. Over time, poor body mechanics become _____ that cause structural deviations.
    a. muscle deviations
    b. repetitive stress injuries
    c. strength exercises
    d. bad postural habits ____

16. When the stress of muscular activity or even gravity is added to a biomechanically weak structure, which of the following results?
    a. dysfunction   c. pain
    b. injury   d. all answers   _____

17. Which of the following aids balance and allows the delivery of firmer, more powerful, more direct massage strokes?
    a. correct posture   c. correct posture and
                               proper foot positions
    b. proper foot positions d. neither correct posture nor
                               proper foot positions   _____

18. The most comfortable stance when doing petrissage on the legs or back is:
    a. archer   c. horse
    b. bear   d. wheel   _____

19. In the horse stance, the shoulders should be:
    a. arched   c. dropped and back
    b. comfortably raised   d. flexed   _____

20. A massage table that is too high may cause:
    a. wrist injury   c. lower back discomfort
    b. shoulder strain   d. neck strain   _____

21. When performing massage, the therapist's shoulders, hips, and feet should be directed toward the:
    a. client's head   c. client's feet
    b. massage table   d. place where the hands are
                               working   _____

22. When applying techniques requiring traction, the practitioner should:
    a. grasp the client   c. put most weight on the
                               front foot
    b. lean back   d. all answers   _____

23. When applying deep pressure, the practitioner should use the hand or arm that is _____ to contact the client and apply pressure.
    a. contra-lateral to the back foot   c. closest to the massage
                                            table
    b. facing away from the client   d. strongest   _____

24. To protect the nerves and other structures passing through the carpal tunnel, angles at the _____ should always exceed 110 degrees.
    a. arm
    b. shoulder
    c. waist
    d. wrist
    _____

25. The practitioner may be seated when working on all of the following body parts *except* the:
    a. back
    b. feet
    c. head
    d. shoulders
    _____

26. The concept that the human body has a geographical center about 2 inches below the navel is called:
    a. centering
    b. grounding
    c. martial arts
    d. spatial massage
    _____

27. The concept that the practitioner has a connection with the client and functions to help the client to release tension is called:
    a. balancing
    b. centering
    c. grounding
    d. shiatsu
    _____

28. *Tan tien* is a Chinese concept referring to:
    a. massage
    b. the body's center
    c. balance
    d. grounding
    _____

29. Being _____ may make you feel insecure and unstable.
    a. centered
    b. confident
    c. negative
    d. uncentered
    _____

30. _____ is achieved by mentally visualizing yourself as having the ability to draw from a greater power or energy.
    a. Body mechanics
    b. Centering
    c. Confidence
    d. Grounding
    _____

31. Which of the following exercises is a movement similar to polishing a car?
    a. archer
    b. grinding corn
    c. horse
    d. wheel
    _____

32. At the beginning of the wheel exercise, the feet should be:
    a. aligned with the massage table
    b. about 6 inches apart
    c. about 12 inches apart
    d. together
    _____

33. In the wheel exercise, what percentage of weight shifts from one foot to the other?
    a. 50   c. 90
    b. 80   d. 100   ____

34. Advance and retreat is a variation of which exercise?
    a. tree   c. wheel
    b. grinding corn   d. archer   ____

35. In advance and retreat, the feet are optimally _____ to _____ inches apart.
    a. 6, 8   c. 12, 18
    b. 12, 14   d. 16, 32   ____

36. In advance and retreat, the primary movement is where?
    a. arms and hands   c. legs and feet
    b. hips and pelvis   d. arms and legs   ____

37. Posture and concentration are emphasized in which exercise?
    a. advance and retreat   c. tree
    b. grinding corn   d. wheel   ____

38. In the tree exercise, it is important to hold the pose for about _____ minutes.
    a. 2   c. 4
    b. 3   d. 5   ____

39. Exercises like grinding corn and wheel improve all of the following *except*:
    a. coordination   c. body weight
    b. proper breathing   d. erect posture   ____

40. The basic rules for safe and effective massage procedures include having nails that are:
    a. short   c. unpainted
    b. painted neutral shades   d. all answers   ____

41. According to the basic rules for safe and effective massage, massage should be avoided:
    a. when the client is fatigued
    b. when the massage room is warm
    c. immediately after the client has eaten a meal
    d. when the client is under stress   ____

42. According to the basic rules of safe massage, the practitioner should never use any form of heavy stroking:
   a. when the client is fatigued
   b. toward the heart
   c. on the client's back
   d. against the venous blood supply

____

Part 3: Massage Practice

CHAPTER 12—PROCEDURES FOR COMPLETE BODY MASSAGES

MULTIPLE CHOICE

1. At the preliminary interview, the therapist should obtain a signed _____ explaining the therapist's services and qualifications.
   a. release of responsibility
   b. release of information form
   c. employee policy manual
   d. informed consent document ____

2. Which of the following is one of the two commonly asked questions about massage?
   a. How long will the massage take?
   b. Where do I leave my belongings?
   c. Do I have to take off my clothes?
   d. Do you offer hydrotherapy? ____

3. What is used to protect client modesty?
   a. personal attention
   b. draping
   c. air conditioning
   d. lubricants ____

4. When clients are lying on their backs, bolsters are placed:
   a. under their necks
   b. under their knees
   c. under their ankles
   d. over their abdomens ____

5. When necessary, _____ may substitute for high-density foam bolsters during massage.
   a. towels
   b. firm bed pillows
   c. electric blankets
   d. stacked books ____

6. Elevating the client's _____ 6 to 8 inches helps the practitioner work on the back more effectively.
   a. abdomen
   b. back
   c. knees
   d. neck ____

7. When a client is in the _____ position, one pillow or cushion is placed under the head to keep the cervical spine straight.
   a. prone
   b. torqued
   c. side-lying
   d. supine ____

8. Which position provides excellent access when working on the inside or outside of the thigh and on the side of the neck?
   a. prone
   b. side-lying
   c. reverse
   d. supine
   _____

9. All bolsters and pillows that directly contact the client must have removable cloth slipcovers that are changed:
   a. for each movement
   b. twice daily
   c. weekly
   d. for each client
   _____

10. All of the following increase the rate at which the body loses heat *except*:
    a. massage lubricant
    b. seated position
    c. perspiration
    d. reclining position
    _____

11. Massage stimulates the _____, affecting the basal body temperature, which chills the client more easily.
    a. kidneys
    b. central nervous system
    c. thyroid
    d. parasympathetic nervous system
    _____

12. If the massage room is cooler than _____ degrees F, extra precautions should be taken to ensure the client stays warm.
    a. 72
    b. 75
    c. 78
    d. 80
    _____

13. Which draping method uses a table covering with a top covering large enough to cover the entire body?
    a. table covering
    b. full sheet
    c. top cover
    d. dressing area
    _____

14. In the top-cover draping method, when the client is lying on the table, two towels are placed in a(n) _____-shaped configuration.
    a. A
    b. L
    c. S
    d. T
    _____

15. In the full-sheet draping method, a full-size, double flat sheet at least _____ inches wide covers the table and wraps the client.
    a. 60
    b. 75
    c. 80
    d. 100
    _____

16. In the massage practice, clean linens must be used:
    a. daily   c. for each movement
    b. for each client   d. weekly   _____

17. In the top-cover draping method, which of the following may be
    used as the top cover?
    a. twin flat sheet   c. large bath sheet
    b. two bath towels   d. all answers   _____

18. Attitudes are often communicated through _____ and
    _____ with people as much as they are through spoken
    words.
    a. interactions, disagreements   c. interest, dealings
    b. actions, physical contact   d. conversations, e-mails   _____

19. Before beginning a professional body massage, it is important to
    _____ the client.
    a. critique   c. tune-in to
    b. bill   d. refer to   _____

20. When the client is in a quiet state of relaxation with the eyes
    closed, the only communication is:
    a. eye contact   c. verbal
    b. written   d. touch   _____

21. The massage sequence can best be defined as:
    a. type of massage performed   c. preparation for a
                                           massage
    b. pattern or design of a massage d. duration of a massage   _____

22. The massage sequence is always _____ enough so that a
    client's individual needs can be addressed.
    a. interesting   c. restricted
    b. demanding   d. flexible   _____

23. When performing massage, the benefits of working from general
    to specific include all of the following except:
    a. decreased spasms   c. decreased circulation
    b. congestion relief   d. ischemic condition relief   _____

24. The final step of a relaxing wellness massage is:
    a. apply effleurage
    b. apply feather strokes
    c. use effleurage to apply lubricant
    d. redrape the massaged body part   _____

25. To apply lubricant efficiently, use _____ to cover the area to be massaged.
    a. petrissage
    b. superficial strokes
    c. tapotement
    d. friction
    _____

26. To have the client breathe deeply and fully, tell the client to breathe through the nose deeply so that which body area expands first?
    a. abdominal
    b. chest
    c. mouth
    d. nose
    _____

27. Some clients are uncomfortable with ear massage because:
    a. massage can cause ear infections
    b. the outer ear is very sensitive
    c. the inner ear is sensitive to touch
    d. no answers
    _____

28. Which countries have developed auricular therapies that points of the outer ear are reflexively related to every body area and organ?
    a. England, Spain
    b. India, China
    c. France, China
    d. Germany, Sweden
    _____

29. A massage of the ear begins with which massage stroke?
    a. petrissage
    b. gliding stroke
    c. circular friction
    d. aura stroking
    _____

30. To prepare for massage of the abdominal region, a bolster or pillow should be placed:
    a. behind the client's neck
    b. under the client's hips
    c. behind the client's knees
    d. under the client's ankles
    _____

31. One optional motion used as a finishing touch for a full-body massage is:
    a. neck petrissage
    b. light pressure on the sacrum
    c. a slight rocking motion
    d. gliding to the neck
    _____

32. On the day of an afternoon massage, a client should drink _____ quarts of water.
    a. 1
    b. 2
    c. 4
    d. 0
    _____

33. The aftereffects of massage may include all of the following *except*:
    a. upset stomach
    b. severe headache
    c. slight headache
    d. nausea

    ____

Part 3: Massage Practice

CHAPTER 13—HYDROTHERAPY

MULTIPLE CHOICE

1. The three forms of water include all of the following *except*:
   a. liquid
   b. gel
   c. ice
   d. vapor _____

2. Which of the following is known as the universal solvent?
   a. water
   b. soap
   c. water and soap
   d. neither water nor soap _____

3. Water has the ability to _____ heat.
   a. absorb
   b. conduct
   c. absorb and conduct
   d. neither absorb nor conduct _____

4. Water is used for facials and steam baths in what form?
   a. liquid
   b. solid
   c. vapor
   d. all answers _____

5. Applying water at temperatures above or below body temperature creates which of the following effects?
   a. chemical
   b. mechanical
   c. thermal
   d. therapy _____

6. _____ effects are produced by the pressure exerted on the surface of the body by sprays, whirlpool baths, and friction.
   a. Chemical
   b. Mechanical
   c. Thermal
   d. Therapy _____

7. Buoyancy reduces the weight of an object immersed in water according to the:
   a. weight of the water
   b. temperature of the object
   c. volume of water displaced by the object
   d. all answers _____

8. _____ reduces the force of gravity and makes it possible to move, float, or exercise in a nearly gravity-free environment.
   a. Cryotherapy
   b. Buoyacy
   c. Hyperthermia
   d. Thermotherapy _____

9. The normal core temperature of the human body is _____ degrees F.
   a. 103.0   c. 92.8
   b. 98.6   d. 37.9   ____

10. When water at a temperature different from that of the skin is applied to skin, the water _____ the heat.
    a. transfers
    b. absorbs
    c. transfers or absorbs
    d. neither transfers nor absorbs   ____

11. The difference between water temperature and skin temperature affects which of the following?
    a. connective tissue   c. nerves
    b. blood vessels   d. all answers   ____

12. When a treatment's temperature is the same as body temperature, which of the following results?
    a. stimulation   c. vasodilation
    b. depressed metabolic activity   d. no thermal effects   ____

13. Full-body applications of heat or cold have _____ effects.
    a. local   c. local and systemic
    b. systemic   d. neither local nor systemic ____

14. At a low temperature, water produces what type of body sensation?
    a. rashes   c. goosebumps
    b. striations   d. all answers   ____

15. Whole-body heat application causes all of the following except:
    a. decreased white blood cell count c. profuse perspiration
    b. increased pulse rate   d. fever-like reaction   ____

16. Which of the following is not caused by local heat application?
    a. local reddening
    b. decreased metabolism
    c. slight analgesia
    d. local musculature relaxation   ____

17. The reduction of body temperature caused by full-body cold application is:
    a. vasodilation   c. hyperthermia
    b. hypothermia   d. vasoconstriction   ____

18. Fascia stiffen with which of the following applications?
    a. initial cold
    b. prolonged cold
    c. initial hot
    d. prolonged hot _____

19. Which of the following applications decrease respiration?
    a. initial cold
    b. prolonged cold
    c. initial hot
    d. all answers _____

20. All of the following are contraindications for water treatments involving hot or cold applications *except*:
    a. cardiac impairment
    b. diabetes
    c. lung disease
    d. bladder infection _____

21. Cryotherapy is the application of _____ agents for therapeutic purposes.
    a. cold
    b. hot
    c. hot and cold
    d. neither hot nor cold _____

22. The third sensation during the prolonged application of ice is:
    a. cold
    b. burning
    c. aching
    d. numbness _____

23. In the CBAN acronym for cold sensations, the letter *N* stands for which of the following?
    a. notice
    b. numbness
    c. neuralgia
    d. natural _____

24. In the RICE acronym for first aid treatment, the *I* stands for:
    a. ice
    b. ischemia
    c. intent
    d. injury _____

25. Contrast therapy is the alternate application of:
    a. heat
    b. cold
    c. heat and cold
    d. neither heat nor cold _____

26. Which of the following is an immediate effect of cold applications?
    a. skin relaxes
    b. surface blood vessels dilate
    c. surface blood vessels constrict
    d. nerve sensitivity increases _____

27. Which of the following treat acute joint and nerve inflammation effectively?
    a. hot compresses
    b. ice packs
    c. vasocoolant sprays
    d. immersion baths ____

28. An inexpensive, convenient way to make a reusable ice pack is to freeze one part _____ to two parts water in a sealable plastic bag.
    a. isopropyl alcohol
    b. ice
    c. antifreeze
    d. chemical gel ____

29. Which method of cryotherapy, when applied to the skin, evaporates very quickly, causing rapid skin cooling?
    a. cold compress
    b. ice pack
    c. vasocoolant spray
    d. compressor unit ____

30. Which of the following transfers heat via conduction?
    a. sauna
    b. infrared
    c. ultrasound
    d. immersion bath ____

31. A steam bath transfers heat via:
    a. conduction
    b. convection
    c. radiation
    d. conversion ____

32. Moderately warm applications have all of the following effects *except*:
    a. muscle relaxation
    b. promoted metabolic activity
    c. profuse sweating
    d. blood vessel relaxation ____

33. The choice of modality for heat application depends on:
    a. body part to be treated
    b. condition of body part to be treated
    c. objectives of the application
    d. all answers ____

34. Which of the following is a dry heat modality?
    a. ultrasound
    b. bath
    c. wrap
    d. compress ____

35. A rice pack is an example of a(n) _____ heat modality.
    a. dry
    b. moist
    c. diathermy
    d. ultrasound ____

36. In diathermy, heat is produced by a(n):
    a. element
    b. ionic vibration
    c. bulb
    d. all answers
    _____

37. _____ is a white or colorless waxy solid that is mixed with mineral oil and heated in a special appliance.
    a. Silica gel
    b. Paraffin
    c. Lotion
    d. Essential oil
    _____

38. _____ is a multi-head, horizontal shower used in a wet room where clients receive massages or other spa treatments.
    a. Swiss shower
    b. Water pic
    c. Vichy shower
    d. Sitz bath
    _____

39. The average cool bath or shower should be limited to _____ to _____ minutes.
    a. 1, 2
    b. 3, 5
    c. 4, 8
    d. 10, 15
    _____

40. Clients complaining of unpleasant reactions during hot baths should receive cold compresses to the:
    a. forehead
    b. back of the neck
    c. forehead and back of the neck
    d. neither forehead nor back of the neck
    _____

41. The first step in a procedure for an immersion bath is:
    a. fill the tub
    b. check room temperature
    c. test water temperature
    d. sanitize the tub
    _____

42. Which bath is often ordered by physicians as part of physical therapy for such conditions as arthritis, sprains, and strained muscles?
    a. immersion
    b. neutral
    c. whirlpool
    d. sitz
    _____

43. A _____ is constructed in an upright or reclining position to accommodate the client's body while leaving the head exposed.
    a. sauna
    b. steam bath
    c. bath cabinet
    d. Vichy shower
    _____

44. Contrast therapy baths should always end with immersion in the
    _____ tub.
    a. hot
    b. cold
    c. hot and cold
    d. neither hot nor cold   ____

Part 3: Massage Practice

CHAPTER 14—MASSAGE IN THE SPA SETTING

MULTIPLE CHOICE

1. The most comprehensive, worldwide spa association, which originated in 1991, is:
   a. Day Spa Association
   b. International Spa Association
   c. Medical Spa Association
   d. Spa Canada
   _____

2. In ancient Rome, the earliest spas were often found at sites to which natural spring water was redirected via:
   a. spa lines
   b. spa services
   c. hammams
   d. aqueducts
   _____

3. The original derivation of the term *spa* is most likely from the Latin verb *spagere*, which means to:
   a. protect
   b. sprinkle
   c. grow
   d. speak
   _____

4. During the height of the Roman empire, the average citizen used _____ gallons of water per day.
   a. 50
   b. 100
   c. 200
   d. 300
   _____

5. The larger ancient Roman baths could accommodate how many people?
   a. 10 to 50
   b. 100
   c. hundreds
   d. thousands
   _____

6. Turkish steam baths, called _____, were part of many mosques until they achieved their own architectural and cultural significance.
   a. thermae
   b. onsen
   c. hammams
   d. banias
   _____

7. The word *hammam* means _____ in Arabic.
   a. spreader of warmth
   b. spring water
   c. hot bath
   d. water for health
   _____

8. Japanese _____ feature baths of varying temperature and treatments, including massage and hydrotherapy.
   a. bania
   b. hammams
   c. onsen
   d. thermae
   ____

9. The German word *kur* came to be synonymous with *spa* in the 1800s when _____ christened his new healing system by that name.
   a. Mary Nelson
   b. Sebastian Kneipp
   c. Mel Zuckerman
   d. Rene Gattfosse
   ____

10. The Native American enclosure in which participants pour water over heated stones to create heat while praying and chanting is a(n):
    a. kiva
    b. onsen
    c. sweat lodge
    d. thermae
    ____

11. The first modern spa that focused on holistic health was the _____, which opened in California in the late 1950s.
    a. Golden Door
    b. Canyon Ranch
    c. Esalen Lodge
    d. Joy Spring Day Spa
    ____

12. According to the 2007 Spa Industry report, there were how many U.S. spas in 2007?
    a. 2,674
    b. 5,500
    c. 14,600
    d. 25,000
    ____

13. Of the spa body services performed at spas in 2007, the most popular was:
    a. hydrotherapy
    b. massage therapy
    c. mud baths
    d. steam baths
    ____

14. Which of the following statements about spa goers is accurate?
    a. Most spa goers are female.
    b. The average age of the spa client is 40.
    c. The average spa goer reports an annual income of over $70,000.
    d. all answers
    ____

15. A spa on a cruise ship is an example of a _____ spa.
    a. destination
    b. day
    c. club
    d. resort
    ____

16. The ancient Indian system of medicine and healing that has been modified in recent years for use in spa treatments is:
    a. kiva
    b. ayurveda
    c. thalassotherapy
    d. aromatherapy   _____

17. Spa employees who pair guests with appropriate treatments, therapists, and services are called intake specialists or:
    a. therapy coordinators
    b. spa therapists
    c. hospitality coordinators
    d. all answers   _____

18. To allow preparation time, it is necessary to end a massage at least _____ minutes before the next treatment is scheduled to begin.
    a. 5
    b. 10
    c. 15
    d. 20   _____

19. At most spas, the typical time frame for a full-body massage is _____ minutes.
    a. 25
    b. 50 to 60
    c. 75 to 80
    d. 90   _____

20. Which of the following is *not* a guideline for greeting spa guests?
    a. Shake hands firmly.
    b. Speak slowly and clearly.
    c. Solicit no tips or gifts.
    d. Offer healthy refreshment during the massage.   _____

21. Hygiene in the treatment room during the day is ultimately the responsibility of the:
    a. spa technician
    b. massage therapist
    c. cleaning crew
    d. intake specialist   _____

22. The term *spa massage* usually refers to what type of massage?
    a. Swedish
    b. Reiki
    c. shiatsu
    d. hydrotherapy   _____

23. Which of the following is *not* a reason it may be challenging for spa therapists to give high-quality, therapeutic massage consistently?
    a. time constraints
    b. low salaries
    c. low expectations
    d. inexperienced clients   _____

24. Which type of massage therapy addresses soft-tissue abnormalities to reduce tightness, pain, and pathologic dysfunction?
    a. Reiki
    b. watsu
    c. wellness/relaxation
    d. neuromuscular
    ____

25. _____ is an ancient massage system that includes stimulation of pressure points and yoga-like stretching to improve health and well-being.
    a. Reiki
    b. Thai massage
    c. Watsu
    d. Shiatsu
    ____

26. Ways to make a spa massage unique include which of the following?
    a. target problem areas
    b. focus on the client's breath
    c. avoid burnout
    d. all answers
    ____

27. In stone massage, stones usually made of _____ are cooled and applied to the skin to complement the effects of heat.
    a. basalt
    b. marble
    c. quartz
    d. slate
    ____

28. One of the most important effects of stone massage derives from its use of alternating hot and cold stones, which is a form of:
    a. contrast therapy
    b. Swedish massage
    c. Reiki
    d. shiatsu
    ____

29. For proper sanitation, massage stones should be cleaned with _____ after each use and before replacement in the heating unit.
    a. alcohol
    b. antibacterial soap
    c. bleach
    d. massage oil
    ____

30. Conditions *not* contraindicated for stone massage but that should have doctor's consent include all of the following *except*:
    a. circulatory problems
    b. high blood pressure
    c. infectious skin disease
    d. Parkinson's disease
    ____

31. In stone massage, stones can be tucked beneath the client's body in such strategic locations as the:
    a. occipital ridge
    b. gluteals
    c. shoulder
    d. all answers
    ____

32. Dry brushing, body polish, and sea salt glow are forms of:
    a. aromatherapy
    c. parafango
    b. exfoliation
    d. watsu
    _____

33. Paraffin wax and fango mud are combined to make _____ for use in spa wraps and localized applications.
    a. fango wax
    c. parafango
    b. paradise mud
    d. spa mud
    _____

34. When water's mineral and gas contents are used therapeutically, it is called:
    a. Scotch hose
    c. watsu
    b. balneotherapy
    d. Vichy shower
    _____

35. Contraindications for the use of the steam bath include all of the following *except*:
    a. diabetes
    c. low blood pressure
    b. hypertension
    d. pregnancy
    _____

36. The use of seawater or sea products (oils, extracts, powders, seaweeds) in baths or other spa treatments is:
    a. balneotherapy
    c. sea salt treatment
    b. exfoliation
    d. thalassotherapy
    _____

37. A(n) _____ uses fans, heat, or steam dispersion to release essential oil aromas into a room for therapeutic and/or esthetic purposes.
    a. aromatherapy
    c. diffuser
    b. carrier
    d. parafango
    _____

38. The word *aromatherapy* was first used in the 1920s by French perfumer:
    a. Mary Nelson
    c. Mel Zuckerman
    b. Rene Gattfosse
    d. Milton Trager
    _____

39. _____ is massage lubricant into which essential oils are blended for aromatherapy applications.
    a. Aromatherapy
    c. Diffuser
    b. Carrier oil
    d. Emulsion
    _____

40. When kept out of direct sunlight and stored in a cool, dry place, essential oils can have a shelf life of:
    a. several days
    c. 3 to 6 months
    b. two weeks
    d. several years
    _____

41. Essential oils that last the longest and are often sweet smelling and calming are categorized as _____ notes.
    a. base
    b. top
    c. center
    d. middle
    _____

42. The style of massage developed in northern California featuring long, flowing strokes that connect all body parts into a whole is:
    a. Swedish massage
    b. shiatsu
    c. Esalen massage
    d. thalassotherapy
    _____

43. Which of the following essential oils derives from a leaf?
    a. lavender
    b. neroli
    c. jasmine
    d. eucalyptus
    _____

44. How many drops of essential oil should be added to each ounce of carrier oil before use in aromatherapy massage?
    a. 12 to 15
    b. 20 to 30
    c. 65
    d. 120
    _____

45. Which diffuser turns liquid oils into an extremely fine mist that fills an area with scent?
    a. atomizer
    b. clay diffuser
    c. fan diffuser
    d. light bulb ring
    _____

46. Which type of body wrap is used to purge and draw impurities out through the pores, softening the skin?
    a. mud
    b. seaweed
    c. mud and seaweed
    d. neither mud nor seaweed
    _____

47. Common characteristics of body wraps include all of the following except:
    a. warmth
    b. comfort and security
    c. essential oils
    d. enclosed environment
    _____

48. A _____ is a thin, transparent, disposable plastic sheet used to wrap directly around a client's skin during mud body wraps.
    a. plastic body wrap
    b. space blanket
    c. thermal blanket
    d. hydrocollator
    _____

49. Hot springs or baths, especially the baths of ancient Rome, are termed:
    a. bania
    b. thermae
    c. hammam
    d. kiva
    _____

50. The root of the word *exfoliation* comes from the Latin *folium*, meaning:
    a. lift
    b. leaf
    c. skin
    d. form _____

51. Which of the following exfoliation procedures is a somewhat rare spa service that can be quite abrasive?
    a. loofah scrub
    b. Swedish shampoo
    c. body gommage
    d. sea salt glow _____

52. A massage room used for spa treatments performed without showers and baths is a:
    a. Vichy shower
    b. dry room
    c. wet room
    d. Swiss shower _____

53. The sea salt glow often uses salts from _____, which are high in such minerals as magnesium, potassium, and calcium.
    a. France
    b. Rome
    c. the Dead Sea
    d. Eastern Europe _____

54. _____ most commonly causes tension between therapists and spa managers.
    a. Compensation
    b. Time management
    c. Customer relations
    d. Physical job demands _____

55. The basic techniques to help the therapist sell spa products tactfully and successfully include all of the following *except*:
    a. self-observation
    b. closing
    c. detachments
    d. commissions _____

56. Anticipating others' needs is what type of skill used by the massage therapist in the spa setting?
    a. sales
    b. teamwork
    c. treatment
    d. professional development _____

57. The massage therapist's first step when pursuing a career in the spa industry is:
    a. be prepared to work on call
    b. create a resume
    c. emphasize customer service skills in interviews
    d. get recommendations from previous employers _____

58. The massage therapist who wants to move up in the spa industry should do all of the following *except*:
    a. always work independently
    b. become active
    c. learn from others
    d. lay a foundation
    ____

59. The massage therapist who decides to open a spa should first:
    a. start slowly
    b. enlist allies
    c. assess limitations
    d. all answers
    ____

Part 3: Massage Practice

CHAPTER 15—CLINICAL MASSAGE TECHNIQUES

MULTIPLE CHOICE

1. A clear idea of what you are trying to accomplish is called:
   a. purpose
   b. intent
   c. technique
   d. knowledge   ____

2. _____ therapies assess tissues and deliver soft tissue manipulative techniques to reprogram the neurological loop.
   a. Mechanical
   b. Massage
   c. Neurophysiological
   d. Anatomical   ____

3. All of the following are examples of neurophysiological therapies *except*:
   a. hydrotherapy
   b. muscle energy techniques
   c. myofascial techniques
   d. trigger-point therapy   ____

4. Stanley Leif and _____ developed the system of soft tissue manipulation called neuromuscular therapy.
   a. Boris Chaitow
   b. Judith DeLany
   c. Raymond Nimmo
   d. James Vannerson   ____

5. Raymond Nimmo and James Vannerson developed what they called _____, which treated "noxious nodules" in hypertonic muscles.
   a. Neuromuscular Therapy
   b. Trigger Point Therapy
   c. Position Release Techniques
   d. Receptor Tonus Technique   ____

6. _____ worked to develop effective neuromuscular protocols for use by soft tissue therapists.
   a. David Simons
   b. Judith Walker
   c. Leon Chaitow
   d. Janet Travell   ____

7. In 1996, _____ published *Modern Neuromuscular Techniques*.
   a. Leon Chaitow
   b. Judith DeLany
   c. Stanley Leif
   d. Paul St. John   ____

8. The body continuously endures stresses from which of the following?
   a. improper nutrition
   b. poor posture
   c. trauma
   d. all answers _____

9. Neuromuscular changes cause all of the following *except*:
   a. depression
   b. fatigue
   c. increased mobility
   d. pain _____

10. Careful and systematic examination of the muscle and associated soft tissue identifies such abnormal signs as:
    a. trigger points
    b. tissue congestion
    c. edema
    d. all answers _____

11. Neuromuscular therapy (NMT) treatment involves:
    a. assessment
    b. soft tissue manipulation
    c. assessment and soft tissue manipulation
    d. neither assessment nor soft tissue manipulation _____

12. Injury in its acute inflammatory phase of healing may last _____ to _____ hours or more.
    a. 24, 48
    b. 36, 72
    c. 48, 72
    d. 48, 96 _____

13. The letter *I* in the RICE acronym for soft tissue first aid stands for:
    a. immobilize
    b. ischemia
    c. ice
    d. injury _____

14. Which of the following is the final step in DeLany's four-step therapy protocol for chronic pain conditions?
    a. Restore endurance with conditioning exercises.
    b. Decrease ischemia and trigger points in the soft tissue.
    c. Rebuild strength with exercise and weight training.
    d. Restore flexibility with joint mobilization and passive stretching. _____

15. According to _____ law, the anterior or ventral roots of the spinal nerves are motor and the posterior or dorsal roots are sensory.
    a. Hilton's
    b. Bell's
    c. Facilitation
    d. Arndt-Schultz _____

16. _____ explains how stimuli that activate only nonnociceptive nerves can inhibit pain.
    a. Bell's law
    b. Gate control theory
    c. Law of facilitation
    d. Hilton's law
    ____

17. Deep gliding strokes are applied:
    a. with the palm of the hand
    b. in the direction of underlying muscle fibers
    c. with the finger tips
    d. all answers
    ____

18. Which of the following techniques is sometimes called muscle stripping?
    a. stretching
    b. trigger point therapy
    c. ischemic compression
    d. deep gliding
    ____

19. In ischemic compression, the duration of the pressure is _____ to _____ seconds.
    a. 4, 8
    b. 8, 12
    c. 10, 15
    d. 15, 20
    ____

20. _____ stretching is valuable in overcoming the contractures and neuromuscular programming that restrict mobility.
    a. Active
    b. Deep
    c. Ischemic
    d. Passive
    ____

21. In neuromuscular therapy, which of the following is performed first?
    a. trigger point therapy
    b. stretching
    c. gliding
    d. palpation
    ____

22. Travell and Simons classify trigger points according to their:
    a. pressure response
    b. location
    c. pressure response and location
    d. neither pressure response nor location
    ____

23. A(n) _____ trigger point prevents full lengthening of muscles and refers pain when digitally compressed.
    a. active myofascial
    b. latent myofascial
    c. central
    d. satellite
    ____

24. A(n) _____ trigger point in one muscle may activate a satellite trigger point in another muscle.
    a. associate
    b. attachment
    c. central
    d. primary
    ____

25. Which type of trigger point is believed to be caused by the continuous tension of the taut band caused by a central trigger point?
    a. associate
    b. attachment
    c. latent myofascial
    d. satellite
    ____

26. Which of the following may activate trigger points?
    a. joint dysfunction
    b. arthritic conditions
    c. emotional stress
    d. all answers
    ____

27. The _____ is a self-perpetuating, dysfunctional, neurological circuit.
    a. trigger point end plate
    b. physiopathological reflex arc
    c. gate control theory
    d. trigger point deactivator
    ____

28. Under pressure, trigger points exhibit referred pain or other sensations to _____ that clients often recognize.
    a. acupuncture points
    b. input areas
    c. latent trigger points
    d. target zones
    ____

29. Palpation allows the therapist to recognize which of the following?
    a. constricted tissue
    b. fibrotic tissue
    c. hyperirritable nodule
    d. all answers
    ____

30. In _____ palpation, the skin and subcutaneous tissue move over fibrous muscle tissue to detect ropey or fibrous conditions beneath.
    a. flat
    b. pincer
    c. flat and pincer
    d. neither flat nor pincer
    ____

31. Which of the following modalities did Travell and Simons find most effective at relieving trigger-point activity?
    a. dry needling
    b. agent injection
    c. acupuncture
    d. spray and stretch technique
    ____

32. Which of the following is a method of passively moving a body part toward the body's preference and away from pain?
    a. position release
    b. muscle energy technique
    c. ischemic compression
    d. trigger point pressure release

    _____

33. Ischemic compression was popularized in a technique called Myotherapy by:
    a. Paul St. John
    b. Janet Travell
    c. Bonnie Prudden
    d. Leon Chaitow

    _____

34. Ischemia around central trigger points is addressed with repeated _____ to increase circulation to, and flush, the area.
    a. compression
    b. effleurage
    c. palpation
    d. stretching

    _____

35. In position release technique, reaching a position for trigger point release lowers the trigger point's sensitivity by _____ to _____ percent.
    a. 25, 30
    b. 30, 50
    c. 50, 75
    d. 70, 100

    _____

36. The preferred technique for returning a muscle to its resting length is:
    a. gentle stretching
    b. position release
    c. muscle energy technique using the antagonist
    d. ischemic compression

    _____

37. Who is credited with developing modern muscle energy technique?
    a. T.J. Ruddy
    b. Fred Mitchell
    c. Lawrence Jones
    d. Arthur Lincoln Pauls

    _____

38. Postisometric relaxation and reciprocal inhibition are two basic _____ incorporated during MET manipulations.
    a. muscle relaxants
    b. inhibitory reflexes
    c. trigger point therapies
    d. range of motion techniques

    _____

39. All of the following are variations of muscle energy techniques (MET) except:
    a. length of effort
    b. starting position
    c. breath incorporation
    d. height of therapist

    _____

40. What technique incorporates the theory that as soon as an isometric muscle contraction releases the muscle relaxes?
    a. contract relax
    b. antagonist relax
    c. antagonist contract
    d. contract-relax-contract the opposite   _____

41. Which muscle energy technique applies the physiological process known as reciprocal inhibition?
    a. agonist contract
    b. contract-relax-contract the opposite
    c. antagonist contract
    d. contract relax   _____

42. Pulsed muscle energy technique (PMET) is directed at the inhibited muscle to do all of the following *except*:
    a. stimulate weakened muscle
    b. decrease circulation
    c. facilitate proprioceptive re-education
    d. further inhibit the opposing hypertonic muscle   _____

43. A natural neuromuscular process known as _____ causes muscle fibers related to injured fibers to shorten to protect injured areas.
    a. reciprocal inhibition   c. proprioception
    b. triggering   d. splinting   _____

44. Which of the following variations of muscle energy technique helps reduce fibrosis in the muscle fascia?
    a. isolytic
    b. pulsed
    c. contract-relax-antagonist-contract
    d. reciprocal inhibition   _____

45. Which technique is also known as passive positioning technique?
    a. ischemic compression   c. position release
    b. neuromuscular therapy   d. muscle energy technique _____

46. Which position release technique is also known as the "tender point" technique?
    a. orthobionomy
    b. strain-counterstrain
    c. structural/muscular balancing
    d. no answers   _____

47. English osteopath Arthur Lincoln Pauls developed which position release technique?
    a. orthobionomy
    b. strain-counterstrain
    c. structural/muscular balancing
    d. reciprocal inhibition   _____

48. It is *not* accurate to say that muscles in a hypertonic state:
    a. contain trigger points
    b. generally are ischemic
    c. may be painful
    d. have low nerve activity   _____

49. Fascicles are arranged alongside one another to form muscles held in place by the:
    a. endomysium   c. myofascia
    b. epimysium   d. perimysium   _____

50. The viscous gel _____, which is as much as 70 percent water, provides the medium for connective tissue fibers and cells.
    a. fibroblast   c. elastin
    b. collagen   d. ground substance   _____

51. Weblike _____ fibers form the framework of some organs and glands and provide support around smooth muscle and nerves.
    a. collagen   c. reticular
    b. elastin   d. fibroblast   _____

52. The connective tissue cells known as _____, which are part of the immune system, synthesize antibodies.
    a. macrophanges   c. mast cells
    b. plasma cells   d. fibroblasts   _____

53. Via _____, hyaluronic acid in connective tissue's ground substance shifts from a gel state to a more fluid one.
    a. thixotrophy   c. tensegrity
    b. piezoelectricity   d. inhibition   _____

54. _____ is the characteristic of certain materials to create and conduct electrical current under pressure or stress.
    a. Thixotrophy   c. Piezoelectricity
    b. Hydrotherapy   d. Tensegrity   _____

55. Myofascial techniques are directed toward which type of fascia?
    a. superficial
    b. deep
    c. superficial and deep
    d. neither superficial nor deep ____

56. Restricted myofascia is indicated through such imbalances in body posture as:
    a. protracted head
    b. tilted pelvis
    c. elevated ilium
    d. all answers ____

57. Tension or resistance found during fascial glide indicates fascial restrictions that may be the result of:
    a. ischemia
    b. fibrous cross-linking
    c. dehydration of the ground substance
    d. all answers ____

58. Which technique is used in chronic or late subacute stages of tissue healing to break down adhesions that may hinder mobility?
    a. muscle rolling
    b. cross-fiber friction
    c. J-stroke
    d. cross-handed stretch ____

59. The intention of indirect myofascial techniques is to:
    a. unlock restrictions
    b. lengthen muscle
    c. unlock restrictions and lengthen muscle
    d. neither unlock restrictions nor lengthen muscle ____

60. The _____ system includes the meninges, cerebrospinal fluid, and the physiological structures that control fluid input and outflow.
    a. fascial
    b. myofascial
    c. craniosacral
    d. cerebral ____

61. The layer of the meninges that is highly vascularized and provides nutrients to nervous tissue is the:
    a. dura mater
    b. pia mater
    c. spinal column
    d. arachnoid membrane ____

Part 3: Massage Practice

CHAPTER 16—LYMPH MASSAGE

MULTIPLE CHOICE

1. Johannes Asdonk published a report on the effects, indications, and contraindications of lymph drainage massage in:
   a. 1932
   b. 1967
   c. 1976
   d. 1987 _____

2. In many parts of Europe today, doctors recommend lymph drainage massage to manage:
   a. stress
   b. lymphedema
   c. high blood pressure
   d. all answers _____

3. Before starting to study lymph massage, the practitioner or student must have thorough knowledge of:
   a. anatomy
   b. kinesiology
   c. physiology
   d. all answers _____

4. Whereas blood circulation is a closed loop, lymph circulation is:
   a. open
   b. two way
   c. one way
   d. no answers _____

5. Lymph circulation ends when lymph re-enters the venous blood flow in an area called the:
   a. angulus venosus
   b. lymph capillary
   c. collector
   d. precollector _____

6. The lymphatic system is made up of:
   a. lymph
   b. lymph nodes
   c. lymph vessels
   d. all answers _____

7. The walls of _____ are composed of one layer of flat, endothelial cells.
   a. collectors
   b. trunks
   c. lymph ducts
   d. lymph capillaries _____

8. Once inside the capillaries, fluid from the interstitial spaces is considered:
   a. chyle
   b. lymph
   c. axillary
   d. all answers _____

9. Lymph is carried from the capillaries to the slightly larger:
   a. collectors
   b. pre-collectors
   c. bicuspid valves
   d. trunks _____

10. The cloudy liquid that passes from the small intestines, through the lacteals, and into the lymph system is called:
    a. chyle
    b. lymph
    c. lacteal
    d. lymphocyte _____

11. The walls of _____ are several cells thick and contain smooth muscle that helps propel lymph.
    a. collectors
    b. trunks
    c. pre-collectors
    d. nodes _____

12. Interstitial fluid derives from which of the following?
    a. lymph
    b. lacteal
    c. blood plasma
    d. all answers _____

13. Between 80 and 98 percent of waste-containing interstitial fluid does which of the following?
    a. absorbs into the lymphatic system
    b. recycles into lymph
    c. reabsorbs into the blood vessels
    d. flushes out of the system through the kidneys _____

14. All of the following are found in lymph *except*:
    a. fats
    b. hormones
    c. tissue debris
    d. chyle _____

15. Inward or _____ vessels carry contaminated lymph to the lymph nodes.
    a. afferent
    b. efferent
    c. lacteal
    d. vascular _____

16. In the lymph nodes, antigens, damaged cells, and toxins are acted on, broken down, or devoured by the:
    a. lacteals
    b. lymph ducts
    c. lymphocytes
    d. all answers _____

17. Once rendered harmless, toxins pass through the lymph ducts and back into the blood system to be eliminated through the:
    a. digestive system
    b. kidneys
    c. lungs
    d. all answers _____

18. Before re-entering the venous blood system, lymph from the right side of the head and neck flows into the:
    a. left lymphatic duct
    b. right lymphatic duct
    c. right thoracic duct
    d. inguinal lymph node
    _____

19. Which of the following is *not* a factor inhibiting lymph flow?
    a. fatigue
    b. surgical lymph node removal
    c. increased physical activity
    d. emotional trauma
    _____

20. The major node areas that drain superficial lymph include all of the following *except* the:
    a. wrists
    b. sides of the neck
    c. inguinal crease
    d. axillary area
    _____

21. Which of the following is *not* a main function of the lymph nodes?
    a. monocyte production
    b. toxin filtration
    c. lymphocyte destruction
    d. lymph concentration
    _____

22. Regional lymph nodes beneath the mandible are considered:
    a. inguinal
    b. popliteal
    c. submaxillary
    d. occipital
    _____

23. _____ nodes are located along the carotid artery and internal jugular vein.
    a. Axillary
    b. Deep cervical
    c. Postauricular
    d. Supratrochlear
    _____

24. Axillary nodes receive lymph from vessels that drain which of the following?
    a. mammary glands
    b. wall of the thorax
    c. upper wall of the abdomen
    d. all answers
    _____

25. B-lymphocytes are produced and mature in the:
    a. thymus gland
    b. bone marrow
    c. spleen
    d. all answers
    _____

26. _____ are produced in the bone marrow and migrate and mature in the thymus.
    a. T-lymphocytes
    b. B-lymphocytes
    c. Antigens
    d. Antibodies
    _____

27. Which of the following is *not* a secondary lymphoid organ?
    a. adenoid
    b. lymph node
    c. thymus
    d. tonsil
    _____

28. It is accurate to say that lymph massage:
    a. increases lymphocyte production
    b. stimulates lymph node activity
    c. improves body metabolism
    d. all answers
    _____

29. All of the following are contraindications of lymph massage *except*:
    a. acne
    b. inflammation
    c. kidney dysfunction
    d. thrombosis
    _____

30. In lymph massage, applied pressure is between _____ and _____ ounces per square inch.
    a. 1, 3
    b. 1, 8
    c. 2, 6
    d. 3, 8
    _____

31. Each circular stroke of lymph massage slightly stretches the skin and underlying tissues in an inverted _____ -shaped pattern.
    a. O
    b. S
    c. L
    d. T
    _____

32. Lymph massage is applied using all of the following *except* the:
    a. fingers
    b. palm
    c. thumb
    d. knuckles
    _____

33. In lymph massage, each movement is repeated in the same area at least _____ to _____ times.
    a. 2, 3
    b. 3, 5
    c. 4, 6
    d. 5, 10
    _____

34. Lymph massage of the arms begins where?
    a. axillary area
    b. hands
    c. arms
    d. pectoral area
    _____

35. For lymph massage on the back of the lower leg, movements are directed toward the:
    a. inguinal crease
    b. axillary area
    c. popliteal space
    d. all answers
    _____

36. For lymph massage of the neck, the practitioner should be:

a. standing on the side being massaged
b. seated above the client's head
c. standing at the head of the table
d. standing on the right side of the table _____

37. Massage of the upper quadrant begins where?
    a. axillary area
    b. pectoral area
    c. arms
    d. breasts _____

38. Lymph massage of the upper quadrants ends where?
    a. axillary area
    b. base of the neck near the angulus venosus
    c. sternal border
    d. popliteal space _____

39. Before performing lymph massage of the inguinal area, the practitioner should:
    a. obtain the client's informed consent
    b. move to a seated position
    c. massage the anterior legs
    d. undrape the client _____

40. A watershed is the separation of lymph flow into the:
    a. inguinal crease
    b. different drainage territories
    c. lower quadrant
    d. greater trochanter _____

41. Lymph massage on the medial half of the posterior thigh begins at the:
    a. popliteal space
    b. inguinal crease
    c. gluteal crease
    d. axillary area _____

42. Lymph massage should finish with:
    a. massage of the scalp
    b. effleurage to the inguinal area
    c. relaxing neck and shoulder massage
    d. gentle massage of the lower back _____

Part 3: Massage Practice

CHAPTER 17—THERAPEUTIC PROCEDURE

MULTIPLE CHOICE

1. Therapeutic procedure is the process of:
   a. acquiring a concise medical history
   b. developing treatment plans
   c. performing appropriate treatment practices
   d. all answers _____

2. The final step in therapeutic procedure is:
   a. assessment   c. performance
   b. evaluation   d. planning _____

3. In which step of the therapeutic procedure does the therapist determine strategies and select therapeutic techniques to address conditions?
   a. assessment   c. performance
   b. evaluation   d. planning _____

4. The therapeutic process is valuable for:
   a. conducting massage sessions   c. long-range goal setting
   b. short-range planning   d. all answers _____

5. In long-range goal setting, the assessment might be extensive and the planning may encompass _____ to _____ sessions.
   a. 3, 5   c. 6, 10
   b. 4, 8   d. 8, 12 _____

6. Which of the following is true of short-range planning?
   a. client's needs are considered
   b. treatment strategy is decided
   c. indications and contraindications are determined
   d. all answers _____

7. According to a 2007 Caravan Opinion Research survey, 22 percent of respondents received massage to:
   a. improve some health concern
   b. relax or reduce stress
   c. relieve pain
   d. pamper themselves _____

8. During the preliminary interview, mirroring the client with a similar voice tone and posture help to:
   a. establish rapport
   b. assess client needs
   c. prevent miscommunication
   d. all answers   ____

9. Which of the following is essential to determining clients' needs and concerns?
   a. length of preliminary interview
   b. clear communication
   c. length of preliminary interview and clear communication
   d. neither length of preliminary interview nor clear communication   ____

10. Client feedback should be encouraged _____ the session.
   a. before   c. during
   b. after   d. all answers   ____

11. The client intake process for therapeutic massage differs from that for wellness/relaxing massage in that the former:
   a. is less extensive
   b. is more extensive
   c. begins with informed consent
   d. no answers   ____

12. Policies and procedures are explained during which segment of the client intake process?
   a. appointment setting   c. assessment
   b. initial consultation   d. informed consent   ____

13. Special tests like range of motion are conducted during which stage of the client intake process?
   a. assessment   c. treatment plan
   b. informed consent   d. initial consultation   ____

14. Common assessment protocol includes all of the following *except*:
   a. close observation
   b. palpation
   c. referral to another health professional
   d. medical history   ____

15. A client information form may include questions about the client's:
    a. age
    b. occupation
    c. reasons for seeking massage services
    d. all answers ____

16. A medical history form includes all of the following information about the client *except*:
    a. past surgeries
    b. reason for seeking massage services
    c. major illnesses
    d. allergies ____

17. The practitioner/client interview is clients' opportunity to:
    a. complete medical history forms   c. tell their stories
    b. explain massage procedures   d. all answers ____

18. Which of the following is an appropriate medical health history question regarding a painful condition?
    a. When did the injury occur?
    b. Can you describe the pain?
    c. How did the condition start?
    d. all answers

19. A client's description of ongoing lower back pain is an example of which type of information?
    a. subjective   c. performance
    b. objective   d. intake ____

20. On a subjective pain scale of 0 to 10, excruciating pain has a rating of:
    a. 1   c. 5
    b. 2   d. 10 ____

21. On a subjective pain scale of 0 to 10, the pressure with the greatest therapeutic value has a client rating of:
    a. 2   c. 7
    b. 5   d. 9 ____

22. The Arndt-Schultz law states that strong stimuli _____ physiological processes.
    a. activate   c. increase
    b. inhibit   d. manipulate ____

23. Visual observation gives the therapist an assessment of:
    a. structural alignment
    c. variations in skin color
    b. bilateral discrepancies
    d. all answers
    ____

24. Observing posture gives many indications of:
    a. structural deviation
    b. muscular imbalance
    c. structural deviation and muscular imbalance
    d. neither structural deviation nor muscular imbalance
    ____

25. When assessing posture, note symmetry of the body's bony landmarks, including all of the following *except* the:
    a. ears
    c. iliac crests
    b. neck
    d. fibular heads
    ____

26. Where should an assessment of posture begin?
    a. feet
    c. AC joints
    b. ears
    d. elbows
    ____

27. Postural distortion may result from which of the following?
    a. pathologic conditions
    c. age
    b. poor work habits
    d. all answers
    ____

28. Compensation for postural deviation usually increases tension on:
    a. connective tissue
    b. postural muscle
    c. connective tissue and postural muscle
    d. neither connective tissue nor postural muscle
    ____

29. A pattern or manner of walking is known as:
    a. posture
    c. posture and gait
    b. gait
    d. neither posture nor gait
    ____

30. Dr. James Cyriax clarified concepts that are invaluable when assessing range of motion, including all of the following *except*:
    a. inert tissue
    c. end feel
    b. capsular patterns
    d. cardiac tissue
    ____

31. Which of the following is an example of contractile tissue?
    a. tendons
    c. bursa
    b. blood vessels
    d. all answers
    ____

32. Nerves are an example of:
    a. inert tissue
    c. capsular patterns
    b. contractile tissue
    d. muscle tissue
    ____

33. The change in movement quality near the end of movement is known as:
    a. contractile pattern
    c. joint limitation
    b. end feel
    d. capsular pattern   _____

34. End feel plays a very important part in assessing _____ movement.
    a. active
    c. active and passive
    b. passive
    d. neither active nor passive _____

35. _____ end feel is an abrupt, painless limitation to movement at the normal end of range of motion, such as knee extension.
    a. Hard
    c. Springy
    b. Soft
    d. Empty   _____

36. When contractile tissues are involved in muscle testing, which type of movement gives a positive result?
    a. active
    c. active and resisted
    b. resisted
    d. neither active nor resisted _____

37. Which type of barrier represents the limits within which tissues can be effectively manipulated?
    a. anatomical
    c. resistive
    b. physiologic
    d. soft tissue   _____

38. Moving beyond the anatomical barrier may cause which of the following?
    a. bruised or damaged tissue
    b. activation of latent trigger points
    c. injury to motor endplates
    d. all answers   _____

39. The pliable and easily movable range of tissue is known as:
    a. freely flexible range of movement
    b. range of motion
    c. soft tissue barrier
    d. springy end feel   _____

40. _____ is the means of communication between the therapist and the client's body.
    a. Body language
    c. End feel
    b. Touch
    d. Medical history   _____

41. Assessment by palpation is:
    a. objective
    b. subjective
    c. objective and subjective
    d. neither objective nor subjective ____

42. In superficial palpation, cool areas may indicate:
    a. increased activity   c. increased circulation
    b. inflammation   d. congestion ____

43. In descriptive terms, the opposite of chronic is:
    a. acute   c. diffuse
    b. circumscribed   d. rigid ____

44. The site of superficial lymph nodes and blood vessels is the:
    a. skin surface
    b. superficial fascia
    c. epimysium
    d. skeletal muscles ____

45. A common palpable muscle condition that is usually associated with a lesion is a:
    a. taut band   c. ropelike tendon
    b. tendon sheath   d. pliable muscle ____

46. A lingering or an ongoing condition is called:
    a. chronic   c. acute
    b. deep   d. superficial ____

47. In the TART assessment protocol, the final letter *T* stands for:
    a. tissue   c. tenderness
    b. texture   d. temperature ____

48. The focus of inflammatory response is _____ of the damaged tissues.
    a. repair
    b. reorganization
    c. repair and reorganization
    d. neither repair nor reorganization ____

49. During what stage of inflammatory response do fibroblasts generate the collagen fibers that bind tissues?
   a. acute
   b. regenerative
   c. remodeling
   d. chronic
   _____

50. Which of the following may be included in a treatment plan?
   a. referral to another health professional
   b. areas of the body to be avoided
   c. recommendations for home self-care
   d. all answers
   _____

51. During the performance of a massage, a visual assessment will note all of the following *except*:
   a. body position
   b. color of the area
   c. symmetry
   d. texture of the skin
   _____

52. Constrictions in soft tissue usually result from all of the following *except*:
   a. body trauma
   b. emotional stress
   c. overuse
   d. underuse
   _____

53. The second step of soft-tissue intervention is:
   a. Release trigger points and fascial restrictions in the muscle tissue.
   b. Rebuild strength and endurance in the muscle.
   c. Relieve inflammation.
   d. Restore circulation and neuromuscular response to the tissues.
   _____

54. Postural muscles have a higher proportion of which type of muscle fibers?
   a. I
   b. II
   c. III
   d. IV
   _____

55. When a muscle is constricted and overactive, it is common for the antagonist to be:
   a. hypertonic
   b. hypotonic
   c. tight
   d. deviated
   _____

56. Which of the following techniques increases local circulation?
   a. stripping
   b. superficial gliding
   c. contrast therapy
   d. all answers
   _____

57. Which of the following would be part of a treatment plan for a client whose treatment goal is to reduce ischemia?
    a. skin rolling
    b. stripping
    c. hydrotherapy
    d. all answers

    _____

58. A palpable tissue response to therapeutically applied pressure is known as:
    a. inhibition
    b. fibrosis
    c. rebound
    d. resistance

    _____

59. Which of the following is *not* one of the three goals of therapeutic massage?
    a. eliminating trigger points
    b. restoring contractile muscle tissue to normal resting length
    c. decreasing muscle tonicity
    d. reducing fibrosis

    _____

60. _____ helps determine whether goals have been met and whether referral to another professional is warranted.
    a. Assessment
    b. Evaluation
    c. Production
    d. Planning

    _____

Part 3: Massage Practice

CHAPTER 18—ATHLETIC/SPORTS MASSAGE

MULTIPLE CHOICE

1. Jack Meagher and Pat Boughton published the first book on sports massage in the United States in:
   a. 1966   c. 1980
   b. 1972   d. 1984   ____

2. Sports massage was first made available for all athletes competing in the summer games at the:
   a. 1984 Olympics in Los Angeles
   b. 1980 Olympics in Stockholm
   c. 1980 Olympics in Lake Placid
   d. 1972 Olympics in Munich   ____

3. The professional sports teams that employ professional massage therapists as part of their training staff include:
   a. baseball   c. hockey
   b. football   d. all answers   ____

4. Athletic massage, also called sports massage, is the application of specific massage skills and knowledge of:
   a. strength training
   b. physiological systems
   c. strength training and physiological systems
   d. neither strength training nor physiological systems   ____

5. Massage helps to reduce the chance of injury by identifying and eliminating conditions in the _____ that are at risk of injury.
   a. epidermis   c. lymph system
   b. soft tissue   d. all answers   ____

6. Adaptive sports massage is available to all athletes with physical disabilities except those with:
   a. amputations   c. high blood pressure
   b. hearing impairments   d. no answers   ____

7. A pre-event massage done on a sprinter with cerebral palsy would be considered:
   a. invigorating
   b. stimulating
   c. relaxing
   d. all answers
   _____

8. Structural deviations often appear as patterns of:
   a. injury
   b. integrated movement
   c. structural balance
   d. structural imbalance
   _____

9. The principle of forcing the body to adapt to heavier loads by increasing strength or endurance is known as:
   a. biomechanics
   b. overload
   c. tensegrity
   d. integration
   _____

10. Among the negative effects of exercise is increased:
    a. endurance
    b. metabolic waste buildup
    c. strength
    d. all answers
    _____

11. It normally takes a muscle stressed to the point of fatigue _____ to _____ hours to rest, adapt, and recuperate.
    a. 12, 24
    b. 24, 36
    c. 36, 48
    d. 48, 72
    _____

12. Massage stretches and broadens which of the following?
    a. muscles
    b. tendons
    c. ligaments
    d. all answers
    _____

13. Many athletic massage techniques are identical to those in _____ massage.
    a. Swedish
    b. shiatsu
    c. acupuncture
    d. hydrotherapy
    _____

14. Which of the following causes increased amounts of blood to remain in the muscle over an extended period?
    a. neuromuscular techniques
    b. compression strokes
    c. lymph massage
    d. myofascial techniques
    _____

15. Hyperemia is beneficial in which type of massage?
    a. restorative
    b. rehabilitative
    c. pre-event
    d. all answers
    _____

16. The release of histamines and acetylcholine causes which of the following?
    a. dilation of blood vessels
    b. softening of adhesions
    c. broadening of muscle tissue
    d. all answers   ____

17. Deep pressure strokes for athletic massage are usually applied with all of the following *except* the:
    a. thumb   c. palm
    b. braced finger   d. elbow   ____

18. Trigger point pressure release technique is another name for:
    a. deep pressure
    b. ischemic compression
    c. deep pressure and ischemic compression
    d. neither deep pressure nor ischemic compression   ____

19. Trigger points that produce pain only when pressure is applied are called:
    a. active   c. referred
    b. latent   d. satellite   ____

20. The massage technique applied by rubbing across tendon, muscle, or ligament fibers at a 90-degree angle is:
    a. cross-fiber friction   c. lymph massage
    b. deep compression   d. shaking   ____

21. When shaking a limb, it is important to avoid:
    a. applying traction to the arm
    b. hyperextending any joint
    c. applying traction to the arm and hyperextending any joint
    d. neither applying traction to the arm nor hyperextending any joint ____

22. In the 1950s, _____ developed active movement exercises for the rehabilitation of conditions like spinal cord injuries and polio.
    a. Margaret Knott   c. Herman Kabat
    b. Dorothy Voss   d. James Cyriax   ____

23. Active stretching movements used in athletic massage borrow from the principles of:
    a. proprioceptive neuromuscular facilitation
    b. muscle energy technique
    c. neuromuscular technique
    d. no answers   ____

24. Which technique is based on reciprocal inhibition and post-isometric relaxation?
    a. neuromuscular technique
    b. proprioceptive neuromuscular facilitation
    c. deep compression
    d. muscle energy technique ____

25. Which athletic massage application is used after an event to normalize tissues and relax the athlete?
    a. restorative   c. rehabilitative
    b. post-event   d. all answers ____

26. _____ massage, which is delivered at the site of an athletic event, is designed to help athletes prepare for or recover from event participation.
    a. Event   c. Restorative
    b. Rehabilitative   d. Integrative ____

27. Pre-event massage is which of the following?
    a. fast paced
    b. invigorating
    c. fast paced and invigorating
    d. neither fast paced nor invigorating ____

28. Which of the following statements about pre-event massage is *false*?
    a. Pre-event massage is a replacement for a warm-up.
    b. Pre-event massage uses no lubricant.
    c. Pre-event massage causes hyperemia.
    d. Pre-event massage is usually given through the clothing. ____

29. The main goals of intra-event massage include all of the following *except*:
    a. help the tissues prepare for an upcoming event
    b. encourage quick recovery from the previous activity
    c. address soft tissue injury
    d. address areas of tension that developed during the event ____

30. Which of the following questions can be used in the post-event massage to determine the athlete's state of mind?
    a. Where would you like me to focus?
    b. How do you feel about your performance?
    c. Have you had something to drink?
    d. How did your training go? ____

31. The pre-event prone - back/upper body massage ends with which technique?
    a. effleurage strokes
    c. compression
    b. light tapotement
    d. circular friction _____

32. When performing a scapula release, bring the arm above the head and apply traction for _____ to _____ seconds.
    a. 2, 3
    c. 10, 12
    b. 5, 7
    d. 12, 15 _____

33. In the prone - lower body procedure, which technique is performed on the gastrocnemius?
    a. petrissage
    b. compression
    c. petrissage and compression
    d. neither petrissage nor compression _____

34. To perform the quadriceps stretch portion of the supine - lower body procedure, the athlete should be positioned:
    a. supine
    c. prone
    b. side-lying
    d. seated _____

35. Chest and arm massage ends with which of the following?
    a. petrissage on the forearms
    b. effleurage up the arm
    c. range of motion for the shoulder
    d. shaking of the arm _____

36. The benefits of training massage include all of the following except:
    a. increased lymph circulation
    b. decreased blood circulation
    c. more efficient metabolic waste removal
    d. decreased chance of injury _____

37. In restorative massage, fascial restrictions are addressed with myofascial techniques that include all of the following except:
    a. broad plane releases
    c. compression
    b. skin rolling
    d. traction _____

38. When treating ankle strains, the therapist should use the thumb and forefinger to apply _____ to the stress points near the ankle bone.
    a. cross-fiber friction
    b. pressure
    c. cross-fiber friction and pressure
    d. neither cross-fiber friction nor pressure _____

39. In athletic massage of the hip area, which of the following is *not* a main stress area?
    a. back of the leg
    b. knee
    c. buttock
    d. side of the hip _____

40. Which of the following activities may injure the wrist ligaments, tendons, or muscles?
    a. bicycling
    b. weight lifting
    c. bicycling and weight lifting
    d. neither bicycling nor weight lifting _____

41. Shoulder joint injuries are often the result of sports like all of the following *except*:
    a. bicycling
    b. basketball
    c. baseball
    d. bowling _____

42. Rehabilitation athletic massage accomplishes which of the following?
    a. reduces edema
    b. deactivates trigger points
    c. increases range of motion
    d. all answers _____

43. Which therapeutic modality is used in rehabilitation massage to control swelling?
    a. lymph massage
    b. myofascial techniques
    c. Swedish massage
    d. neuromuscular techniques _____

44. All of the following are examples of traumatic athletic injuries *except*:
    a. torn ligaments
    b. dislocated joints
    c. broken bones
    d. strained muscles _____

45. Which grade of strain or sprain is characterized by swelling and possible discoloration?
    a. I
    b. II
    c. III
    d. IV _____

46. Which phase of healing for soft tissue injury is also known as the regenerative stage?
    a. acute
    b. early subacute
    c. inflammatory
    d. remodeling _____

47. Myofascial techniques are applied at and around an injury to site help to create a strong, flexible scar during which phase of soft tissue healing?
    a. maturation
    b. acute
    c. chronic
    d. early subacute _____

48. All of the following are examples of chronic injury *except*:
    a. tendonitis
    b. tennis elbow
    c. dislocated shoulder
    d. iliotibial band syndrome _____

49. The delicate connective tissue covering of muscle fibers is the:
    a. endomysium
    b. fascicle
    c. epimysium
    d. sarcolemma _____

50. Which of the following is a positive effect of swelling?
    a. slowed healing
    b. immobilized area
    c. damaged tissue
    d. all answers _____

51. During healing, collagen formation that reconnects the injured tissue forms:
    a. fascia
    b. scar tissue
    c. fibroblasts
    d. fascicles _____

52. Practitioner behavior like imprudent action or failure to take reasonable precautions is considered:
    a. malpractice
    b. contraindications
    c. judgment
    d. negligence _____

Part 3: Massage Practice

CHAPTER 19—MASSAGE FOR SPECIAL POPULATIONS

MULTIPLE CHOICE

1. All of the following are special populations requiring special considerations for massage therapy *except* the:
   a. elderly
   b. sedentary
   c. pregnant
   d. critically ill
   _____

2. Massage during pregnancy is termed _____ massage.
   a. prenatal
   b. natal
   c. perinatal
   d. parenting
   _____

3. During pregnancy, a woman's body experience what type of changes?
   a. hormonal
   b. physical
   c. hormonal and physical
   d. neither hormonal nor physical
   _____

4. All of the following are physical changes caused by pregnancy *except*:
   a. enlarged breasts
   b. lower back strain
   c. frequent mood changes
   d. weight gain
   _____

5. For the pregnant client in the supine position, pillows or a foam wedge should support a _____ position.
   a. reclining
   b. side-lying
   c. semi-reclining
   d. sitting
   _____

6. The supine position is cautioned during the second and third trimesters of pregnancy because the fetus may press on the:
   a. heart
   b. kidneys
   c. sciatic nerve
   d. descending aorta
   _____

7. During pregnancy, massage to the lower back can be applied in the _____ position.
   a. prone
   b. supine
   c. side-lying
   d. all answers
   _____

8. Which of the following is *not* a contraindication of prenatal massage?
   a. high blood pressure
   c. minor edema
   b. decreased fetal movement
   d. morning sickness
   _____

9. Which of the following is a symptom of pre-eclampsia?
   a. edema
   c. sodium retention
   b. high blood pressure
   d. all answers
   _____

10. The effects of progesterone and relaxin on the blood vessels can cause which of the following conditions?
    a. edema
    c. varicose veins
    b. pre-eclampsia
    d. miscarriage
    _____

11. Normal human pregnancy lasts how long?
    a. 7 months
    c. 35 weeks
    b. 40 weeks
    d. 10 months
    _____

12. High risk factors in the first trimester include all of the following *except*:
    a. previous miscarriages
    c. Rh-negative father
    b. maternal age
    d. gestation of twins
    _____

13. What special consideration should be made for massage clients experiencing morning sickness in the first trimester of pregnancy?
    a. focus on rhythmic movements
    b. massage scheduled when symptoms are minimal
    c. focus on abdominal massage
    d. all answers
    _____

14. The second trimester of pregnancy last from weeks _____ to _____.
    a. 3, 12
    c. 12, 24
    b. 8, 16
    d. 14, 26
    _____

15. In the second trimester of pregnancy, the body starts to produce the hormone _____, which softens the pelvis's connective tissues.
    a. relaxin
    b. toxemia
    c. relaxin and toxemia
    d. neither relaxin nor toxemia
    _____

16. In the third trimester of pregnancy, pressure on the _____ causes shortness of breath and hyperventilation.
    a. uterus   c. heart
    b. veins   d. diaphragm   _____

17. _____ are the mild, irregular practice contractions experienced in the third trimester of pregnancy as uterine muscles tense for short periods.
    a. Dilators   c. Relaxins
    b. Braxton-Hicks   d. Stress contractions   _____

18. In 1973, Vimala Schneider McClure witnessed infant massage in what country?
    a. Bali   c. India
    b. Nigeria   d. Romania   _____

19. Who founded the International Loving Touch Foundation in 1992?
    a. Diana Moore   c. Frederick Leboyer
    b. Vimala Schneider McClure d. Tiffany Field   _____

20. A person or persons whose responsibility is rearing a child is called a:
    a. prenatal consultant   c. child proxy
    b. primary care giver   d. no answers   _____

21. All of the following are benefits of infant massage except:
    a. bonding
    b. inhibition of the digestive system
    c. relief of tension and pain
    d. relaxation   _____

22. During infant massage, a sleeping baby indicates:
    a. relaxation   c. disengagement
    b. engagement   d. a successful treatment   _____

23. An acceptable choice of massage lubricant for infant massage is _____ oil.
    a. grapeseed   c. sweet almond
    b. olive   d. all answers   _____

24. The infant massage routine for colic ends with which of the following?
    a. clockwise petrissage   c. circular friction
    b. jostling friction   d. effleurage   _____

25. In the Well Baby Massage Routine for the head and face, which body part is massaged first?
    a. forehead
    c. nose
    b. jaw
    d. scalp   _____

26. An elderly person with limited vitality and age-associated illness is considered:
    a. vital
    c. frail
    b. robust
    d. challenged   _____

27. For clients with auditory impairments, massage considerations include all of the following *except*:
    a. tapping the client on the shoulder
    b. reading nonverbal clues like twitching
    c. pointing to communicate
    d. providing mobility aids   _____

28. Which of the following is *not* a mobility aid?
    a. crutches
    c. walker
    b. service dog
    d. wheelchair   _____

29. A stroke or cerebral vascular accident may paralyze one side of the body, which is known as:
    a. quadriplegia
    c. paraplegia
    b. hemiplegia
    d. tetraplegia   _____

30. Thoracic or lumbar spine injuries paralyze the legs and lower body in a condition called:
    a. wheelchair bound
    c. hemiplegia
    b. paraplegia
    d. quadriplegia   _____

31. Long-term paralysis is often accompanied by:
    a. joint stiffness
    b. muscle atrophy
    c. joint stiffness and muscle atrophy
    d. neither joint stiffness nor muscle atrophy   _____

32. The causative agent for acquired immune deficiency syndrome (AIDS) is:
    a. Candida
    c. Kaposi's sarcoma
    b. human immunodeficiency virus
    d. toxoplasmosis   _____

33. Shingles, an opportunistic infection associated with AIDS, is a form of which virus?
    a. herpes
    c. meningitis
    b. Candida
    d. pneumonia
    ____

34. _____ is cancer of the cells lining certain blood vessels.
    a. Varicella-zoster
    c. Candida albicans
    b. Kaposi's sarcoma
    d. Myeloma
    ____

35. For cancer patients, the benefits of massage include all of the following *except*:
    a. improved flexibility
    c. reduced anxiety
    b. decreased lymph movement
    d. improved elimination
    ____

36. Fewer than _____ percent of metastatic cells from a tumor survive in the bloodstream.
    a. 20
    c. 5
    b. 10
    d. 1
    ____

37. At which stage of metastasis do viable malignant cells reach the capillary bed of a preferred host tissue?
    a. direct invasion
    b. cells breaking off the primary tumor
    c. implantation of cancerous cells at secondary sites
    d. circulation through the blood and lymph vessels
    ____

38. The type of cancer that originates in lymphatic tissue is:
    a. sarcoma
    c. lymphoma
    b. carcinoma
    d. leukemia
    ____

39. Highly abnormal, undifferentiated cancerous cells are considered which grade level?
    a. 1
    c. 3
    b. 2
    d. 4
    ____

40. The stages of cancer quantify which of the following to express the extent of the disease?
   a. status of the primary tumor
   b. regional lymph node involvement
   c. areas of metastasis
   d. all answers _____

41. In Stage _____, cancer is well developed and has spread to other tissues or organs.
   a. I
   b. II
   c. III
   d. IV _____

42. Which of the following notations is used to indicate no evidence of tumor?
   a. NX
   b. N0
   c. T1-4
   d. T0 _____

43. All of the following are common cancer treatments *except*:
   a. steroid administration
   b. radiation
   c. lymph transplant
   d. chemotherapy _____

44. For the massage therapist, surgery increases the chances of which serious consideration?
   a. nausea
   b. thrombus
   c. edema
   d. all answers _____

45. Which of the following is not a side effect of chemotherapy?
   a. nausea
   b. fever
   c. vertigo
   d. increased platelet count _____

46. Reduced red blood cell counts cause anemia, which causes which of the following?
   a. fatigue
   b. cold intolerance
   c. shortness of breath
   d. all answers _____

47. When cancer treatment reduces a client's platelet count, the client may be prone to:
   a. bruising
   b. bleeding
   c. bruising and bleeding
   d. neither bruising nor bleeding _____

48. When _____ are low, a client's immune system may be compromised, making the client more vulnerable to infection.
   a. white blood cells
   b. red blood cells
   c. platelets
   d. all answers _____

49. The term *alopecia* is another name for:
    a. swelling
    b. hair loss
    c. nausea
    d. skin irritation

    _____

50. The medical term for weight loss is:
    a. alopecia
    b. cachexia
    c. neuropathy
    d. pathogenesis

    _____

51. When chemotherapy affects the central or peripheral nervous system, all of the following may result *except*:
    a. burning sensations
    b. pain
    c. intolerance to cold
    d. tingling sensation

    _____

52. Which form of cancer treatment requires tattooing the patient's body?
    a. chemotherapy
    b. bone marrow transplant
    c. radiation
    d. surgery

    _____

53. A client who experiences nausea while undergoing radiation treatment should avoid which of the following?
    a. passive movement techniques
    b. rocking
    c. joint movements
    d. all answers

    _____

54. For clients with cancer, massage sessions should be adjusted to the:
    a. cancer
    b. cancer treatment
    c. client's level of health
    d. all answers

    _____

55. In the hospice setting, patients generally have prognoses of:
    a. disease remission
    b. less than 6 months to live
    c. cancer recurrence
    d. 6 months of rehabilitation

    _____

56. Hospice patients generally tolerate no more than _____ to _____ minutes of touch.
    a. 5, 10
    b. 10, 15
    c. 15, 20
    d. 25, 30

    _____

57. Which type of energy work may help hospice patients accept death as part of life?
    a. Therapeutic Touch
    b. Reiki
    c. Therapeutic Touch and Reiki
    d. neither Therapeutic Touch nor Reiki

    _____

Part 3: Massage Practice

CHAPTER 20—MASSAGE IN MEDICINE

MULTIPLE CHOICE

1. There is evidence that the Greeks employed massage-like treatments for medical purposes in the times of:
   a. Rhazes
   b. Hippocrates
   c. Avicenna
   d. Mercurialis
   ____

2. By the sixteenth century in the West, medical practitioners again began using:
   a. exercise
   b. gymnastics
   c. mechanotherapy
   d. all answers
   ____

3. Per Henrik Ling's system of medical gymnastics became known as the _____ Cure.
   a. Movement
   b. Swedish
   c. Movement or Swedish
   d. neither Movement nor Swedish
   ____

4. Who completed full training in the Movement Cure at the Sotherberg Institute in Stockholm before returning to New York?
   a. Charles Fayette Taylor
   b. Mary McMillan
   c. Douglas Graham
   d. George Henry Taylor
   ____

5. In 1902, _____ published *Manual Therapies, A Treatise on Massage.*
   a. Mary McMillan
   b. Douglas Graham
   c. James Mennell
   d. Charles Fayette Taylor
   ____

6. Until about 1945, massage for treating _____ conditions continued to expand in the United States.
   a. stress
   b. chronic
   c. lymphatic
   d. orthopedic
   ____

7. English osteopaths Stanley Lief and Boris Chaitow developed:
   a. trigger point therapy
   b. Neuromuscular Technique (NMT)
   c. cross-fiber techniques
   d. craniosacral therapy
   ____

8. Techniques that effectively addressed soft tissue conditions in athletes also effectively treated which conditions in the general population?
   a. hypertonic
   b. dysfunctional
   c. hypertonic and dysfunctional
   d. neither hypertonic nor dysfunctional _____

9. _____ medicine treats disease or injury with medications and surgery.
   a. Allopathic
   b. Alternative
   c. Holistic
   d. Integrative _____

10. The term _____ *medicine* replaced the term *alternative medicine* in the 1980s.
    a. allopathic
    b. complementary
    c. holistic
    d. integrative _____

11. The acronym CAM stands for _____ medicine.
    a. complementary allopathic
    b. complementary and alternative
    c. collective allopathic
    d. no answers _____

12. Which of the following is considered a CAM modality?
    a. humor therapy
    b. hydrotherapy
    c. chiropractic
    d. all answers _____

13. Which of the following terms means to look at the whole picture?
    a. holistic
    b. integrative
    c. alternative
    d. complementary _____

14. Which of the following is *not* considered a mind-body technique?
    a. guided imagery
    b. nutrition
    c. meditation
    d. yoga _____

15. Integrative medicine combines allopathic medicine with which of the following types of medicine?
    a. complementary
    b. alternative
    c. complementary and alternative
    d. neither complementary nor alternative _____

16. An Eisenberg study showed that, in 1997, Americans spent more than _____ dollars on alternative therapies.
    a. 300 million
    b. 562 billion
    c. 825 million
    d. 27 billion _____

17. According to a 2007 survey, conditions for which CAM was most often used included all of the following *except*:
    a. headaches
    b. insomnia
    c. soft tissue injuries
    d. joint pain _____

18. When working with chiropractors on clients with soft tissue injuries, massage therapists will do all of the following *except*:
    a. deactivate trigger points
    b. increase circulation
    c. reduce spasms
    d. adjust joints _____

19. On top of the list of treatments for patients using integrative medicine is:
    a. meditation
    b. yoga
    c. massage
    d. chiropractic _____

20. Which type of massage reduces pain and increases range of motion and function to a particular body area?
    a. lymph drainage massage
    b. orthopedic massage
    c. shiatsu
    d. craniosacral therapy _____

21. In the hospital setting, the therapist may be required to demonstrate certain competencies using which of the following methods?
    a. verbal exams
    b. written tests
    c. hands-on demonstrations
    d. all answers _____

22. In a hospital setting, the massage therapist must follow hospital regulations for:
    a. patient information
    b. patient safety
    c. record confidentiality
    d. all answers _____

23. What becomes the communication tool between various modalities in the hospital setting?
    a. verbal communication
    b. accurate records
    c. nonverbal communication
    d. all answers _____

24. In the hospital setting, the therapist may not massage a patient without a _____ from a physician.
    a. recommendation
    b. referral
    c. prescription
    d. all answers _____

25. Before a hospital can pursue payment from an insurance company for massage services, what is required?
    a. patient payment
    b. physician's prescription
    c. physician's referral
    d. all answers

    _____

26. In the hospital setting, massage is usually performed:
    a. in the patient's hospital bed
    b. only during morning hours
    c. in a massage room
    d. by a physician

    _____

27. Massage before surgery reduces which of the following?
    a. patient anxiety
    b. recovery time
    c. patient anxiety and recovery time
    d. neither patient anxiety nor recovery time

    _____

28. Arthritis and bursitis are examples of what of condition, which is contraindicated for massage?
    a. varicose veins
    b. inflamed joints
    c. infection
    d. cancer

    _____

29. Which of the following is *not* a warning sign that is associated with cancer and contraindicated for massage?
    a. breast lump
    b. persistent sore throat
    c. skin tag of changed color
    d. excessive edema

    _____

30. It is accurate to say that medical massage:
    a. is prescribed by a physician
    b. may occur in a massage therapist's studio
    c. is performed to treat medically diagnosed conditions
    d. all answers

    _____

31. Which of the following is a diagnosed condition that is referred for medical massage?
    a. osteoarthritis
    b. carpal tunnel syndrome
    c. athletic injury
    d. all answers

    _____

32. Proper billing for insurance reimbursement requires all of the following *except*:
    a. accurate record keeping
    b. SOAP method of record keeping
    c. clear communication with the company agent
    d. close attention to detail when preparing claims

    _____

33. Which of the following insurance coverage types is most likely to cover massage therapy?
    a. Worker's Compensation
    c. Medicaid
    b. PPO
    d. Medicare
    _____

34. For insurance verification purposes, the client's insurance ID number is often the same as the:
    a. Social Security number
    c. claim number
    b. policyholder's name
    d. CPT code
    _____

35. At the time of service, the patient must pay which of the following?
    a. service fee
    c. co-pay
    b. reimbursement
    d. disbursement
    _____

36. On a doctor's prescription, the prescribed treatment is the:
    a. ICD-9
    c. claim number
    b. license number
    d. CPT code
    _____

37. When speaking with an insurance adjuster, which of the following might the therapist ask about the deductible?
    a. How many sessions are allowed?
    b. When does the deductible renew?
    c. How much time is allowed per treatment per diagnosis?
    d. all answers
    _____

38. Which form allows the carrier to send claim benefits directly to the therapist for services performed?
    a. Agreement for Payment Form
    b. Assignment of Benefits Form
    c. Medical Information Release Form
    d. Intake Form
    _____

39. The _____ form may be part of the Intake Form or a separate document.
    a. Assignment of Benefits
    c. Informed Consent
    b. Initial Assessment
    d. Medical History
    _____

40. The Health Care Financing Administration created the _____ form so service providers could bill insurance for medical expenses.
    a. 1500 Health Insurance Claim
    c. Agreement for Payment
    b. SOAP
    d. CMS
    _____

41. In SOAP documentation, the letter *P* stands for:
    a. prognosis   c. physician
    b. plan   d. palpatory   ____

42. CPT codes are arranged according to:
    a. medical specialty
    b. injury location
    c. medical specialty and injury location
    d. neither medical specialty nor injury location   ____

43. The CPT code for manual traction is:
    a. 97010   c. 97140
    b. 97124   d. 1500   ____

44. CPT codes change how often?
    a. annually   c. monthly
    b. daily   d. weekly   ____

Part 3: Massage Practice

CHAPTER 21—ADDITIONAL THERAPEUTIC MODALITIES

MULTIPLE CHOICE

1. Which type of massage is found in airports, shopping malls, and supermarkets?
   a. acupuncture
   b. chair
   c. Feldenkrais
   d. all answers
   ____

2. All of the following modalities regularly work with clients in a seated position *except* the:
   a. Rolfing
   b. Trager method
   c. Feldenkrais
   d. Alexander technique
   ____

3. Chair massage was formulated and popularized by:
   a. Charles Fayette Taylor
   b. Stanley Lief
   c. David Palmer
   d. Bruno Chikly
   ____

4. Today, most bodywork schools include some form of _____ in their core curricula.
   a. chair massage
   b. Reiki
   c. shiatsu
   d. Feldenkrais
   ____

5. For those with negative touch experiences, chair massage is a way to reintroduce which of the following?
   a. bodywork techniques
   b. body centering
   c. emotional touch
   d. positive touch
   ____

6. The average cost of a weekly table massage is $_____ to $_____.
   a. 5, 15
   b. 25, 40
   c. 45, 60
   d. 50, 80
   ____

7. Chair massage is the easiest way to experience massage for the first time because it is:
   a. easy to learn
   b. lacking in contraindications
   c. low cost
   d. all answers
   ____

8. Chair massage students can begin their practice massages sooner than other therapists because chair massage:
   a. takes less time than table massage
   b. is easier to learn than table massage
   c. is very versatile
   d. requires no formal study   _____

9. All of the following body parts are readily accessible to chair massage therapists *except* the:
   a. back   c. abdomen
   b. neck   d. hips   _____

10. The massage chair's face cradle and armrest should be sanitized after each use with:
    a. an antimicrobial wipe   c. bleach
    b. soap and water   d. hand sanitizer   _____

11. A seated client may experience a sudden drop in blood pressure, which may lead to symptoms of:
    a. edema   c. heart disease
    b. back ache   d. fainting   _____

12. Seated clients commonly faint or experience symptoms of fainting due to:
    a. low blood sugar
    b. history of fainting
    c. low blood sugar and history of fainting
    d. neither low blood sugar nor history of fainting   _____

13. Which of the following is *not* a sign that a client may be about to faint?
    a. nausea   c. sudden sweating
    b. headache   d. lightheadedness   _____

14. Chair massage should end with which of the following massage techniques?
    a. compression   c. circular friction
    b. nerve strokes   d. light hacking   _____

15. _____ is based on the principles that reflex points in the hands and feet are related to every body organ and area.
    a. Swedish massage   c. Reflexology
    b. Chair massage   d. Lymph massage   _____

16. The roots of reflexology date back over 4,000 years with painted hieroglyphs in ancient:
    a. China
    b. Rome
    c. Egypt
    d. India
    _____

17. Western reflexology began as which of the following?
    a. shiatsu
    b. watsu
    c. zone therapy
    d. acupuncture
    _____

18. *Stories the Feet Can Tell* was written by _____, who furthered the popularity of reflexology.
    a. Joe Riley
    b. Eunice Ingham
    c. David Palmer
    d. William Fitzgerald
    _____

19. During reflexology, the therapist can effect beneficial changes in a distant but related area of the body by applying pressure to:
    a. a reflex point
    b. a trigger point
    c. the thumbs
    d. the sacrum
    _____

20. During a reflexology session, the practitioner feels for inconsistencies and sensitive areas in the:
    a. hands
    b. feet
    c. ears
    d. all answers
    _____

21. When performing reflexology on the foot, the practitioner might need to switch hands to:
    a. reach the bottom of the foot
    b. keep the wrist straight
    c. perform a thumbwalk
    d. all answers
    _____

22. Acupuncture originated in China more than _____ years ago.
    a. 500
    b. 1,000
    c. 5,000
    d. 10,000
    _____

23. The traditional Chinese medical practice whereby the skin is punctured with very thin needles at specific points is:
    a. reflexology
    b. acupuncture
    c. Reiki
    d. shiatsu
    _____

24. In Eastern philosophy, *yin* and *yang* are the parts of the:
    a. chakras
    b. reflex
    c. chi
    d. *tao*
    _____

25. *Yin* and *yang* are seen as _____ of the same phenomenon and exist only in relation to one another.
    a. opposites
    b. problems
    c. opposites and problems
    d. neither opposites nor problems   ____

26. When *yang* is excessive, *yin* is:
    a. active
    b. deficient
    c. overactive
    d. all answers   ____

27. In Eastern thought, the inner body is represented by:
    a. *yin*
    b. *yang*
    c. *tao*
    d. no answers   ____

28. When *yin* and *yang* are in balance, the result is:
    a. pain
    b. disharmony
    c. disease
    d. well-being   ____

29. When *yin* and *yang* become severely imbalanced, they separate, causing:
    a. illness
    b. death
    c. fear
    d. anxiety   ____

30. The vital life force of all living matter is known as:
    a. bioforce
    b. bioenergy
    c. bioforce and bioenergy
    d. neither bioforce nor bioenergy   ____

31. Which of the following is *not* one of five interrelated aspects of energy manifested by *chi*?
    a. water
    b. metal
    c. air
    d. wood   ____

32. The meridian *chi* has 12 bilateral meridians, or channels, that are associated with:
    a. respiration
    b. organs
    c. digestion
    d. lymph flow   ____

33. The meridian *chi* has small areas of high conductivity called:
    a. *chi*
    b. needles
    c. acupoints
    d. pressure points   ____

34. Which of the following organ meridians is classified with the earth element?
    a. lung
    b. spleen
    c. liver
    d. kidney
    _____

35. Which of the following organ meridians is classified as *yang*?
    a. stomach
    b. large intestine
    c. gallbladder
    d. all answers
    _____

36. The starting point of the large intestine organ meridian is the:
    a. chest
    b. bottom of the foot
    c. medial side of the eye
    d. index finger
    _____

37. The gallbladder organ meridian is classified as:
    a. wood
    b. yin
    c. fire
    d. water
    _____

38. Acupressure is often used with which of the following?
    a. herbs
    b. diet
    c. meditation
    d. all answers
    _____

39. The Japanese word meaning pressure of the fingers or digits is:
    a. *ki*
    b. *tsubo*
    c. *chi*
    d. *shiatsu*
    _____

40. The purpose of shiatsu is to:
    a. increase circulation
    b. restore energy balances
    c. increase circulation and restore energy balances
    d. neither increase circulation nor restore energy balances
    _____

41. The circular energy centers that move much like mini tornados are called:
    a. *tsubo*
    b. chakras
    c. *chi*
    d. shiatsu
    _____

42. Which of the following may be used to open and balance chakras?
    a. crystals
    b. pendulums
    c. crystals and pendulums
    d. neither crystals nor pendulums
    _____

43. All of the following are energy techniques *except*:
    a. yoga
    b. polarity therapy
    c. Reiki
    d. Touch for Health
    _____

44. Ayurvedic massage is an example of which technique?
    a. energy
    b. manipulative
    c. aromatherapy
    d. movement

    _____

Part 4: Massage Business Administration

CHAPTER 22—MASSAGE BUSINESS ADMINISTRATION

MULTIPLE CHOICE

1. The self-employed massage business person acts as:
   a. owner
   b. bookkeeper
   c. maintenance person
   d. all answers ____

2. Keeping records, understanding laws and regulations, and being familiar with insurance requirements are all part of:
   a. advertising information
   b. business procedures
   c. customer relations
   d. all answers ____

3. Employees may be paid by the hour or by:
   a. commission
   b. minute
   c. flat fee
   d. no answers ____

4. Which of the following is *not* an advantage of being employed by a massage facility?
   a. provide personal equipment
   b. regular paycheck
   c. employee benefits
   d. regular schedule ____

5. Which of the following is a possible employment situation for the massage therapist?
   a. spas
   b. athletic clubs
   c. hospitals
   d. all answers ____

6. Where should the massage therapist check for employment advertisements?
   a. online
   b. local newspaper classifieds
   c. online and local newspaper classifieds
   d. neither online nor local newspaper classifieds ____

7. A(n) _____ should indicate why a prospective employee wants to work for a company.
   a. cover letter
   b. resume
   c. affiliation
   d. work history ____

8. A list of association memberships should appear in what part of a resume?
   a. contact information
   c. qualifications
   b. education
   d. affiliations
   ____

9. The prospective employee should state the position of interest in which section of the cover letter?
   a. intro
   c. work history
   b. body
   d. close
   ____

10. Before the interview, the prospective employee should visit the business's:
   a. web site
   b. location
   c. web site and location
   d. neither web site nor location
   ____

11. At a job interview, candidates should be prepared to answer questions about all of the following *except*:
   a. career goals
   b. personal benefits to the company
   c. health history
   d. qualifications
   ____

12. Which of the following does *not* look professional?
   a. minimal jewelry
   b. discreet gum chewing for fresh breath
   c. clean, polished shoes
   d. well-groomed hair
   ____

13. Within 24 hours after an interview, the prospective employee should:
   a. call the interviewer
   c. visit the company again
   b. send a thank-you letter
   d. no answers
   ____

14. A good self-image and positive attitude are the foundations for creating a good:
   a. business record
   c. massage education
   b. clientele list
   d. public image
   ____

15. All of the following are true of independent contractors *except* that independent contractors:
   a. determine their own work schedules
   b. provide their own supplies
   c. are responsible for their own taxes
   d. are paid hourly
   ____

16. Setting personal work hours is an example of which Internal Revenue Service criteria?
    a. financial control
    b. relationship with the business
    c. behavioral control
    d. client base

    _____

17. Which type of massage therapist may be expected to sign a non-compete agreement?
    a. employee
    b. independent contractor
    c. employee and independent contractor
    d. neither employee nor independent contractor

    _____

18. Massage therapists who work from home:
    a. may need special variances
    b. can provide child care while working
    c. need no waiting areas
    d. all answers

    _____

19. In a(n) _____ setup, a landlord prepares the work space and all supplies.
    a. outcall
    b. home-based office
    c. turnkey situation
    d. co-op

    _____

20. Which massage practice option provides attractive office space while keeping overhead low?
    a. outcalls
    b. co-op
    c. outcalls and co-op
    d. neither outcalls nor co-op

    _____

21. Business planning involves which of the following?
    a. determining priorities
    b. setting goals
    c. stating a mission
    d. all answers

    _____

22. A specific, attainable, measurable thing a person commits to achieve is a:
    a. mission
    b. purpose
    c. goal
    d. passion

    _____

23. The statement "I will make a positive difference for my clientele" is an example of a:
    a. goal
    b. mission
    c. purpose
    d. passion

    _____

24. Which of the following helps clarify intentions and direct creative energy toward realizing dreams?
    a. goal
    b. mission
    c. purpose
    d. passion

    _____

25. For which of the following business types are the practitioner and the business one and the same in the eyes of the law?
    a. co-op
    b. sole proprietorship
    c. Limited Liability Company
    d. all answers ____

26. A business setup in which two or more partners share responsibility and benefits of running the business is a:
    a. sole proprietorship
    b. corporation
    c. partnership
    d. Limited Liability Company ____

27. Which business setup shields owners from some of their businesses' personal liability?
    a. sole proprietorship   c. corporation
    b. partnership   d. Limited Liability Company ____

28. All of the following are examples of professional fees *except*:
    a. business coach   c. Web designer
    b. brochures   d. accountant ____

29. Hiring an attorney is an example of which type of start-up expense?
    a. professional fee   c. advertising
    b. initial operating   d. license and permit ____

30. Which of the following is a factor to consider when buying an established business?
    a. facility
    b. business reputation
    c. projected income and expenses
    d. all answers ____

31. Which of the following may be issued after a business has been inspected and found free of hazards to personnel and clients?
    a. planning permit   c. building safety permit
    b. massage license   d. business license ____

32. Which of the following do partnerships and businesses that hire employees need?
    a. employer's identification number (EIN)
    b. fictitious name statement (DBA)
    c. provider's number
    d. sales tax permit ____

33. A business that sells products needs which of the following?
    a. provider's number
    b. massage license
    c. employer's identification number (EIN)
    d. sales tax permit _____

34. An identification number issued to licensed health care providers is called a(n):
    a. employer's identification number (EIN)
    b. provider's number
    c. fictitious name statement (DBA)
    d. no answers _____

35. Which type of insurance is also known as malpractice insurance?
    a. professional liability   c. liability
    b. disability   d. property _____

36. Which type of insurance covers the medical costs for employees injured on the job?
    a. professional liability   c. renter's
    b. health   d. worker's compensation _____

37. Which of the following does *not* reflect ethical behavior by a massage therapist?
    a. maintaining good health habits
    b. charging fair price for services
    c. recommending a maximal number of treatments
    d. keeping accurate client records _____

38. Which of the following is an example of nontaxed income?
    a. out-of-state sales   c. wholesale sales
    b. freight   d. all answers _____

39. Which of the following is *not* an expense category for the disbursement ledger?
    a. charitable donations   c. owner's salary
    b. automobile expenses   d. insurance premiums _____

40. For tax reasons, the business owner should keep all receipts for at least _____ years.
    a. 3   c. 7
    b. 5   d. indefinitely _____

41. A record of moneys owed to a party by other persons or businesses is called a(n):
    a. disbursement ledger
    b. accounts receivable
    c. profit and loss statement
    d. accounts payable

42. All business travel in an automobile should be recorded in a(n):
    a. profit and loss statement
    b. asset and depreciation record
    c. appointment book
    d. mileage log

43. Marketing activity that is done in return for direct payment is:
    a. advertising
    b. promotion
    c. advertising and promotion
    d. neither advertising nor promotion

44. The two main sources of referrals are current clients and:
    a. former clients
    b. other health care professionals
    c. advertisements
    d. former employees

45. All of the following are parts of the business bookkeeping system *except*:
    a. petty cash
    b. inventory
    c. business loans
    d. client files

APPENDIX I—BASIC PHARMACOLOGY FOR MASSAGE THERAPISTS

MULTIPLE CHOICE

1. On the intake form, the client should provide which of the following information regarding drug use?
   a. frequency
   b. duration
   c. dosage
   d. all answers
   _____

2. All drugs do which of the following?
   a. cure illness
   b. cause cellular change
   c. derive from plants
   d. affect the entire body
   _____

3. Drugs with effects limited to one area or body part are considered:
   a. local
   b. systemic
   c. local and systemic
   d. neither local nor systemic
   _____

4. The geriatric population metabolizes and excretes medications _____ than younger adults.
   a. much faster
   b. at the same rate as
   c. much slower
   d. no answers
   _____

5. Most drugs are eliminated through the:
   a. skin
   b. large intestine
   c. liver
   d. kidneys
   _____

6. How does body weight affect drug administration?
   a. Heavier patients require lower dosages.
   b. Heavier patients require higher dosages.
   c. Thinner patients have more adverse side effects.
   d. Drug effects have not been studied on heavy adults.
   _____

7. For _____ drug names, the initial letter is never capitalized.
   a. trade
   b. generic
   c. chemical
   d. scientific
   _____

8. The "catchy" or _____ name of a drug is one the public will remember easily.
   a. trade
   b. generic
   c. chemical
   d. scientific
   _____

9. Pharmaceutical companies lose exclusive rights to patented drugs after how many years?
   a. 5
   b. 8
   c. 15
   d. 17
   ____

10. A drug to reduce pain is an:
    a. analgesic
    b. anti-emetic
    c. anti-inflammatory
    d. antipyretic
    ____

11. Which skin medication is a topical used to soothe or protect the skin?
    a. antipruritic
    b. demulcent
    c. corticosteroid
    d. keratolytic
    ____

12. All of the following are examples of antifungals *except*:
    a. Lamisil
    b. Tinactin
    c. Lotrimin
    d. Lindane
    ____

13. Which of the following is an example of an antibacterial?
    a. Cortaid
    b. Erygel
    c. Zovirax
    d. Monistat
    ____

14. Nonsteroidal anti-inflammatory drugs (NSAIDs) work by inhibiting the synthesis of:
    a. immunodilators
    b. prostaglandins
    c. corticosteroids
    d. histamines
    ____

15. Spondylitis should be treated with which kind of medication?
    a. gout agents
    b. nonsteroidal anti-inflammatory drugs
    c. antacids
    d. corticosteroids
    ____

16. Which type of medication neutralizes gastric hydrochloric acid?
    a. antacids
    b. H2 blockers
    c. proton pump inhibitors
    d. all answers
    ____

17. Which of the following is an antiemetic?
    a. Colace
    b. Levsin
    c. Lomotil
    d. Zofran
    ____

18. Drugs that help break up gas in the GI tract are called:
    a. antiemetics
    b. antiflatulents
    c. anticholinergics
    d. cathartics
    ____

19. Medications used to treat nausea, vomiting, and motion sickness are called:
    a. anticholinergics
    b. antacids
    c. cathartics
    d. antiemetics
    _____

20. The three types of bronchodilators include all of the following *except*:
    a. adrenergics
    b. cholinergics
    c. anticholinergics
    d. xanthine derivatives
    _____

21. Which of the following is a bronchodilator?
    a. Albuterol
    b. Codeine
    c. Cromolyn
    d. Flovent
    _____

22. Zyrtec is an example of which type of medication?
    a. decongestants
    b. mucolytics
    c. antihistamines
    d. corticosteroids
    _____

23. Which medications are used mostly to treat congestive heart failure in which the heart fails to pump properly?
    a. antiarrhythmics
    b. calcium channel blockers
    c. cardiac glycosides
    d. antihypertensives
    _____

24. Tekturna HCT targets the enzyme _____, which can contribute to high blood pressure.
    a. diuretic
    b. prostaglandin
    c. xanthine
    d. renin
    _____

25. Hyperkalemia is a side effect of which type of medication?
    a. angiotensin receptor blockers
    b. ACE inhibitors
    c. antihypertensives
    d. cardiac glycosides
    _____

26. Heparin is an example of which type of medication?
    a. platelet inhibitors
    b. antithrombolytics
    c. antilipemics
    d. antiarrhythmics
    _____

27. The most commonly used diuretic is:
    a. loop
    b. thiazide
    c. osmotic
    d. potassium-sparing
    _____

28. Alpha blockers like Flomax are used to treat which of the following conditions?
    a. benign prostatic hypertrophy (BPH)
    b. hepatitis
    c. gout
    d. angina pectoris
    _____

29. _____ drugs stop the growth and spread of malignant cells.
   a. Osmotic
   b. Tumorigenesis
   c. Antineoplastic
   d. Endocrine
   _____

30. Which antineoplastic drug comes from the bark of the Pacific yew?
   a. alkylating drug
   b. biological response modifier
   c. antimetabolite
   d. placlitaxel
   _____

31. Synthetically produced progesterone drugs are called:
   a. estrogens
   b. progestins
   c. androgens
   d. corpus luteums
   _____

32. Side effects of the fertility drug Clomid include all of the following *except*:
   a. insomnia
   b. ovarian cysts
   c. nausea
   d. multiple pregnancies
   _____

33. Amikin, Garamycin, and Nebcin are examples of which type of anti-infective drug?
   a. cephalosporins
   b. quinolones
   c. tetracyclines
   d. aminoglycosides
   _____

34. Anorexia is a side effect of which type of ant-infective drug?
   a. penicillins
   b. macrolides
   c. sulfonamides
   d. aminoglycosides
   _____

35. Rifadin is an example of which type of drug?
   a. antituberculosis
   b. antiviral
   c. fertility
   d. antifungal
   _____

36. Which antiviral medication is used to treat chicken pox?
   a. neuraminidase inhibitor
   b. acyclovir
   c. interferon
   d. ribavirin
   _____

37. Protease inhibitors, nucleoside reverse transcriptase inhibitors, and nonnucleoside reverse transcriptase inhibitors are examples of:
   a. antivirals
   b. analgesics
   c. antiretrovirals
   d. antiurinary drugs
   _____

38. Which medications enhance the analgesic effect when used with opioids and nonopioids?
   a. antivirals
   b. adjuvants
   c. barbiturates
   d. hypnotics
   _____

39. Lunesta, Ambien, and Sonata are examples of which type of medication?
   a. antidepressants
   b. analgesics
   c. barbiturates
   d. nonbarbiturates

   _____

40. Which drugs, also called neuroleptics, are major tranquilizers?
   a. anxiolytics
   b. anticonvulsants
   c. anticholinergic drugs
   d. antipsychotic drugs

   _____

41. Drugs to treat Alzheimer's disease include all of the following *except*:
   a. Eldepryl
   b. Cognex
   c. Aricept
   d. Exelon

   _____

42. _____ is the system of nutritional recommendations from the Institute of Medicine of the United States National Academy of Sciences.
   a. Recommended Dietary Allowances (RDA)
   b. Dietary Reference Intake (DRI)
   c. RDA and DRI
   d. neither RDA nor DRI

   _____

43. In many European countries, herbal medicine, called _____, is considered mainstream.
   a. botanica
   b. pharmacopeia
   c. phytotherapy
   d. pharmacognosy

   _____

Part I: The History and Advancement of Therapeutic Massage

CHAPTER 1—HISTORICAL OVERVIEW OF MASSAGE

1. c	11. b	21. a	31. c	41. c
2. a	12. a	22. d	32. a	42. b
3. b	13. c	23. b	33. d	43. d
4. b	14. c	24. d	34. b	44. a
5. d	15. b	25. a	35. d	45. a
6. d	16. c	26. a	36. c	
7. a	17. a	27. b	37. a	
8. c	18. b	28. a	38. d	
9. a	19. a	29. b	39. c	
10. b	20. c	30. b	40. a	

CHAPTER 2—REQUIREMENTS FOR THE PRACTICE OF THERAPEUTIC MASSAGE

1. b	8. d	15. c	22. b
2. a	9. a	16. d	23. b
3. b	10. c	17. d	24. d
4. c	11. c	18. b	25. d
5. d	12. d	19. b	26. b
6. c	13. d	20. b	27. c
7. b	14. b	21. c	

CHAPTER 3—PROFESSIONAL ETHICS FOR MASSAGE PRACTITIONERS

1. b	11. d	21. d	31. a	41. c
2. d	12. b	22. a	32. d	42. b
3. a	13. c	23. a	33. b	43. c
4. c	14. b	24. a	34. b	44. b
5. b	15. b	25. c	35. d	45. d
6. d	16. a	26. a	36. b	46. c
7. c	17. c	27. d	37. b	47. c
8. a	18. b	28. d	38. d	48. d
9. d	19. b	29. d	39. a	49. a
10. b	20. b	30. a	40. b	50. b

Part II: Human Anatomy and Physiology

CHAPTER 4—OVERVIEW OF HUMAN ANATOMY AND PHYSIOLOGY

1. a	11. a	21. c	31. b	41. b
2. d	12. c	22. b	32. c	42. d
3. b	13. d	23. d	33. b	43. d
4. c	14. a	24. a	34. b	
5. b	15. d	25. c	35. a	
6. a	16. a	26. c	36. c	
7. b	17. c	27. b	37. b	
8. b	18. a	28. b	38. d	
9. b	19. c	29. a	39. a	
10. c	20. b	30. c	40. a	

CHAPTER 5—HUMAN ANATOMY AND PHYSIOLOGY

1. c	27. a	53. a	79. c	105. b
2. d	28. c	54. d	80. a	106. b
3. a	29. c	55. c	81. b	107. c
4. d	30. b	56. d	82. b	108. c
5. b	31. c	57. b	83. c	109. d
6. a	32. b	58. b	84. b	110. b
7. c	33. c	59. b	85. a	111. c
8. a	34. a	60. b	86. c	112. b
9. d	35. b	61. c	87. d	113. a
10. b	36. c	62. b	88. b	114. c
11. b	37. d	63. d	89. c	115. a
12. a	38. b	64. c	90. b	116. a
13. b	39. b	65. a	91. a	117. b
14. d	40. c	66. b	92. b	118. a
15. b	41. a	67. b	93. d	119. d
16. a	42. a	68. d	94. b	120. b
17. b	43. b	69. c	95. b	121. c
18. b	44. c	70. a	96. c	122. b
19. a	45. b	71. b	97. d	123. c
20. d	46. d	72. c	98. d	
21. c	47. a	73. d	99. c	
22. c	48. c	74. b	100. c	
23. b	49. b	75. b	101. d	
24. c	50. a	76. c	102. c	
25. d	51. b	77. d	103. a	
26. d	52. b	78. b	104. b	

Part III: Massage Practice

CHAPTER 6—EFFECTS, BENEFITS, INDICATIONS, AND CONTRAINDICATIONS OF MASSAGE

1. c	11. c	21. c	31. c	41. b
2. d	12. d	22. b	32. c	42. b
3. c	13. a	23. a	33. c	43. b
4. d	14. b	24. c	34. b	44. b
5. b	15. a	25. c	35. a	45. d
6. c	16. c	26. b	36. b	46. a
7. d	17. c	27. d	37. c	47. d
8. d	18. d	28. b	38. d	48. b
9. c	19. b	29. c	39. b	49. c
10. b	20. d	30. a	40. c	

CHAPTER 7—EQUIPMENT AND PRODUCTS

1. b	11. a	21. d	31. a	41. b
2. d	12. a	22. b	32. c	42. b
3. b	13. c	23. c	33. b	43. b
4. b	14. a	24. b	34. d	44. c
5. a	15. d	25. c	35. a	45. a
6. c	16. d	26. d	36. c	
7. a	17. a	27. d	37. c	
8. d	18. b	28. c	38. b	
9. d	19. d	29. d	39. a	
10. b	20. a	30. b	40. c	

CHAPTER 8—SANITARY AND SAFETY PRACTICES

1. c	11. d	21. d	31. b	41. d
2. a	12. d	22. b	32. d	42. b
3. b	13. b	23. b	33. b	43. a
4. d	14. b	24. b	34. c	
5. d	15. d	25. b	35. d	
6. c	16. b	26. a	36. a	
7. b	17. a	27. b	37. c	
8. c	18. a	28. d	38. a	
9. d	19. a	29. c	39. b	
10. c	20. d	30. c	40. b	

CHAPTER 9—THE CONSULTATION

1. a	11. d	21. c	31. c	41. d
2. b	12. a	22. b	32. d	42. b
3. c	13. c	23. b	33. c	43. b
4. d	14. d	24. b	34. b	44. d
5. d	15. b	25. c	35. a	45. a
6. b	16. a	26. a	36. c	
7. a	17. c	27. d	37. d	
8. c	18. d	28. d	38. b	
9. d	19. c	29. b	39. d	
10. b	20. d	30. d	40. c	

CHAPTER 10—CLASSICAL MASSAGE MOVEMENTS

1. b	11. b	21. d	31. b	41. c
2. c	12. d	22. d	32. a	42. b
3. a	13. d	23. a	33. b	43. c
4. c	14. b	24. c	34. c	44. a
5. c	15. c	25. d	35. b	45. c
6. c	16. d	26. a	36. b	46. a
7. c	17. b	27. c	37. b	47. b
8. b	18. d	28. b	38. d	48. d
9. a	19. b	29. c	39. c	49. c
10. c	20. d	30. a	40. d	

CHAPTER 11—APPLICATION OF MASSAGE TECHNIQUE

1. c	11. a	21. d	31. b	41. c
2. d	12. a	22. d	32. b	42. d
3. a	13. c	23. a	33. c	
4. d	14. a	24. d	34. c	
5. d	15. d	25. a	35. d	
6. b	16. d	26. a	36. b	
7. a	17. c	27. c	37. c	
8. c	18. c	28. b	38. b	
9. b	19. c	29. d	39. c	
10. d	20. b	30. d	40. a	

CHAPTER 12—PROCEDURES FOR COMPLETE BODY MASSAGES

1. d	8. b	15. c	22. d	29. c
2. c	9. d	16. b	23. c	30. c
3. b	10. b	17. d	24. d	31. c
4. b	11. d	18. b	25. b	32. b
5. b	12. a	19. c	26. a	33. b
6. a	13. c	20. d	27. b	
7. c	14. d	21. b	28. c	

CHAPTER 13—HYDROTHERAPY

1. b	11. d	21. a	31. b	41. b
2. a	12. d	22. c	32. c	42. c
3. c	13. b	23. b	33. d	43. c
4. c	14. c	24. a	34. a	44. b
5. c	15. a	25. c	35. b	
6. b	16. b	26. c	36. b	
7. c	17. b	27. b	37. b	
8. b	18. b	28. a	38. c	
9. b	19. d	29. c	39. b	
10. c	20. d	30. d	40. c	

CHAPTER 14—MASSAGE IN THE SPA SETTING

1. b	13. b	25. b	37. c	49. b
2. d	14. d	26. d	38. b	50. b
3. b	15. d	27. b	39. b	51. a
4. d	16. b	28. a	40. d	52. b
5. d	17. c	29. b	41. a	53. c
6. c	18. a	30. c	42. c	54. a
7. a	19. b	31. d	43. d	55. d
8. c	20. d	32. b	44. a	56. b
9. b	21. b	33. c	45. a	57. b
10. c	22. a	34. b	46. a	58. a
11. a	23. b	35. c	47. c	59. d
12. c	24. d	36. d	48. a	

CHAPTER 15—CLINICAL MASSAGE TECHNIQUES

1. b	14. a	27. b	40. a	53. a
2. c	15. b	28. d	41. c	54. c
3. a	16. b	29. d	42. b	55. c
4. a	17. b	30. a	43. d	56. d
5. d	18. d	31. d	44. a	57. d
6. b	19. b	32. a	45. c	58. b
7. a	20. a	33. c	46. b	59. a
8. d	21. d	34. b	47. a	60. c
9. c	22. c	35. d	48. d	61. b
10. d	23. a	36. c	49. b	
11. c	24. d	37. b	50. d	
12. d	25. b	38. b	51. c	
13. c	26. d	39. d	52. b	

CHAPTER 16—LYMPH MASSAGE

1. b	11. a	21. c	31. c	41. c
2. b	12. c	22. c	32. d	42. c
3. a	13. c	23. b	33. d	
4. c	14. d	24. d	34. a	
5. a	15. a	25. b	35. c	
6. d	16. c	26. a	36. b	
7. d	17. d	27. c	37. a	
8. b	18. b	28. d	38. b	
9. b	19. c	29. a	39. a	
10. a	20. a	30. b	40. b	

CHAPTER 17—THERAPEUTIC PROCEDURE

1. d	14. c	27. d	40. b	53. a
2. b	15. d	28. c	41. c	54. a
3. d	16. b	29. b	42. d	55. b
4. d	17. c	30. d	43. a	56. d
5. c	18. d	31. a	44. b	57. b
6. d	19. a	32. a	45. a	58. c
7. b	20. d	33. b	46. a	59. c
8. a	21. c	34. b	47. c	60. b
9. b	22. b	35. a	48. c	
10. d	23. d	36. c	49. b	
11. b	24. c	37. d	50. d	
12. b	25. b	38. d	51. d	
13. a	26. a	39. a	52. b	

CHAPTER 18—ATHLETIC/SPORTS MASSAGE

1. b	13. a	25. b	37. c	49. a
2. a	14. b	26. a	38. c	50. b
3. d	15. d	27. c	39. b	51. b
4. d	16. a	28. a	40. c	52. d
5. b	17. c	29. c	41. a	
6. c	18. c	30. b	42. d	
7. c	19. b	31. b	43. a	
8. d	20. a	32. a	44. d	
9. b	21. b	33. c	45. b	
10. b	22. c	34. b	46. b	
11. d	23. a	35. d	47. a	
12. d	24. d	36. b	48. c	

CHAPTER 19—MASSAGE FOR SPECIAL POPULATIONS

1. b	14. d	27. d	40. d	53. d
2. a	15. a	28. b	41. d	54. d
3. c	16. d	29. b	42. d	55. b
4. c	17. b	30. b	43. c	56. c
5. c	18. c	31. c	44. b	57. c
6. d	19. a	32. b	45. d	
7. c	20. b	33. a	46. d	
8. c	21. b	34. b	47. c	
9. d	22. c	35. b	48. a	
10. c	23. d	36. d	49. b	
11. b	24. a	37. c	50. b	
12. c	25. a	38. c	51. c	
13. b	26. c	39. d	52. c	

CHAPTER 20—MASSAGE IN MEDICINE

1. b	11. b	21. d	31. d	41. b
2. c	12. d	22. d	32. b	42. a
3. a	13. a	23. b	33. a	43. c
4. d	14. b	24. d	34. a	44. a
5. b	15. c	25. d	35. c	
6. d	16. d	26. a	36. d	
7. b	17. c	27. c	37. b	
8. c	18. d	28. b	38. b	
9. a	19. c	29. d	39. d	
10. b	20. b	30. d	40. a	

CHAPTER 21—ADDITIONAL THERAPEUTIC MODALITIES

1. b	11. d	21. b	31. c	41. b
2. b	12. c	22. c	32. b	42. c
3. c	13. b	23. b	33. c	43. a
4. a	14. b	24. d	34. b	44. b
5. d	15. c	25. a	35. d	
6. c	16. c	26. b	36. d	
7. c	17. c	27. a	37. a	
8. b	18. b	28. d	38. d	
9. c	19. a	29. b	39. d	
10. a	20. d	30. c	40. c	

CHAPTER 22—MASSAGE BUSINESS ADMINISTRATION

1. d	11. c	21. d	31. c	41. b
2. b	12. b	22. c	32. a	42. d
3. a	13. b	23. c	33. d	43. a
4. a	14. d	24. a	34. b	44. b
5. d	15. d	25. b	35. a	45. c
6. c	16. c	26. c	36. d	
7. a	17. a	27. d	37. c	
8. d	18. a	28. b	38. d	
9. a	19. c	29. a	39. c	
10. c	20. b	30. d	40. c	

APPENDIX I—BASIC PHARMACOLOGY FOR MASSAGE THERAPISTS

1. d	11. b	21. a	31. b	41. a
2. b	12. d	22. c	32. b	42. b
3. a	13. b	23. c	33. d	43. c
4. c	14. b	24. d	34. b	
5. d	15. b	25. b	35. a	
6. b	16. a	26. b	36. b	
7. b	17. d	27. b	37. c	
8. a	18. b	28. a	38. b	
9. d	19. d	29. c	39. d	
10. a	20. b	30. d	40. d